MW01172906

The Addiction Recovery Workbook

Essential Skills to Overcome Any
Addiction and Prevent Relapse

Linda Hill

i

Table of Contents

The First Step in Taking Back Control of Your Life

Did you know that there's an enormous financial cost to addiction? As a general condition, addiction entails being obsessive or dependent on a particular substance or activity. Alternatively, as a neuropsychological disorder, addiction entails a persistent and intense urge to use a certain substance, regardless of the substantial harm it causes you, along with other negative ramifications. Both these definitions entail a lack of control—over your actions, emotions, and behaviors. If you look at this lack of control in the financial realm, it's easy to see how addiction may incur a large financial cost. When you can't control yourself or how often you use a certain substance, then the monetary cost won't even deter you or cause you any hesitation or doubt. You will spend all that money on your addiction and probably won't bat an eye. On top of that, there's also the cost of health care that's inevitably tied to your addiction. The substance that you abuse probably causes a great deal of damage to your physical and mental health, so your addiction will also incur health care costs. This increases the overall cost of your addiction.

There are several other surprising facts about addiction that can help you understand your condition better and increase your resolve to fight it. Let's explore some of these facts. Other than the financial stress it can cause, addiction can also cause co-occurring disorders, leading you to suffer from more than one health condition at the same time. Addiction is usually linked to anxiety, depression, obsessive compulsive disorder, post-traumatic stress disorder, bipolar personality disorder, and other psychotic disorders. These co-occurring disorders increase your emotional distress and make it even harder for you to combat your addiction since you're simultaneously fighting another mental battle. Your addiction and co-occurring disorder may also feed on one another. When you abuse substances, you may trigger depressive or anxious episodes, which in turn may push you to abuse more substances. So, people with addiction are more likely to develop co-occurring disorders, while people with mental health issues are more likely to develop addiction. It's not certain which comes first, but nevertheless, the end result is increased suffering for you. That's where this book comes in—

you can use the tips and strategies that will be provided to fight your addiction and decrease your emotional distress. Treating your addiction will even have a positive effect on any co-occurring disorders you have.

Another little known fact on addiction is that prescription drugs have a higher fatality rate compared to illegal drugs. If your addiction is to prescription drugs, you may brush it under the rug and tell yourself that it's not that dangerous or that at least you're not addicted to those harder drugs such as cocaine or heroin. At least you're not mixed up in anything illegal. But the surprising truth is that legal pills kill more people than illegal drugs do. News reports usually focus on cocaine, heroin, or meth overdoses, as those make for better headlines, and this may be why you're not aware of the dangers of legal, prescription drugs. The fact is that "three million US citizens and 16 million individuals worldwide have had or currently suffer from opioid use disorder (OUD)" (Huecker et al., 2019). And in 2012, "16,000 deaths occurred in the US at the hands of prescription drugs in total" (VitaNova, 2019). The point of this isn't to lower your perception of the dangers of illegal drugs. Such drugs remain a prevalent and destructive force. The point of this is just to increase your awareness of the real dangers of legal, prescription drugs so that you don't make light of your addiction. If you're addicted to a substance, even if it's a legal and prescribed drug, you must recognize the harm and danger of your condition and take action against it.

Moving along from the little known facts about addiction, let's now do a bit of exploring on the little known facts on addicts. The stereotypical image of an addict is someone who is homeless, unemployed, and begging by the side of the street. Or it may be someone causing a ruckus while they're high, disrupting the peace and causing mayhem. This is how most people view addicts, and the underlying assumption is probably that these addicts opted out of society. This might fit easier into a common person's worldview. Addicts are judged negatively and thus they can't possibly fit normally into society. On the other hand, working people are judged positively and seen as contributors to society. These are two opposite ends of a spectrum, so it's understandable how the common person would choose to see addicts as bums and beggars. But the truth is that most addicts are also working people. Addiction doesn't consider your background or income level, so most people suffering from addiction aren't homeless or unemployed. On the surface, they're probably living very normal lives. However, just because you can portray a healthy life, this doesn't mean that you're really leading a healthy life. You must come to terms with your addiction and begin to challenge and fight it.

On that tangent, one last surprising fact about addiction is that early intervention is more effective than intervening at a rock-bottom moment. You may have gathered from movies, books, and other stories that someone with addiction needs to hit rock-bottom before they're willing to seek treatment. However, there's no need to wait for that to happen. If you know you suffer from addiction, or even if it's in the very beginning stages where you're not convinced you're really addicted or that anything's the matter, it would still be wise of you to take action now. Don't wait until the problem gets bigger and more destructive. Get ahead of it now and prevent any further pain and distress.

These are all surprising facts about addiction that will hopefully increase your resolve to fight your own potential addiction, no matter what stage it's at or how intense your symptoms are. And another thing to clarify here is that you may not be addicted to any one substance. Addiction applies to a wide range of substances and activities. You may be addicted to alcohol, drugs, social media, the internet, and so on. Obviously, being addicted to substances is more harmful than other addictions, as those substances physically enter your body and change its chemistry, but the mental state of being addicted in itself is a distressing thing to experience. So, this book is meant to be helpful to anyone suffering from addiction, no matter what they're addicted to.

If you're suffering from addiction, then you may often experience feelings of helplessness. You may not know what you're experiencing, how to stop yourself, or why this is happening to you. Other than that, you may experience drastic shifts in your mood. You may become enraged when denied access to your addiction, depressed when you're alone without access to your addiction, anxious when you're with others and without access to your addiction, or frustrated when delayed access to your addiction. There are countless possible ways that your addiction may impact your moods and emotions and, going back to your feelings or helplessness, it can be hard to control these changes in mood. Another pain point associated with addiction is a lower quality of relationships. Being addicted to something can significantly harm your relationships with others, as you may consistently prioritize your addiction over your friends and loved ones. These friends and loved ones may even be frequent victims to your mood swings and explosive emotions. And you may begin to neglect and spend less time with them as you start to spend more and more time on your addiction. When you're addicted to something, you may also stay at home more often in order to indulge in your addiction. This not only prevents you from spending quality time with your friends and loved ones, it also prevents you from making any meaningful new connections with others.

All these are side effects of addiction that can significantly lower your quality of life. When you're addicted to something, it can take control of your actions, thoughts, and emotions. Your life will be directed by your urges and desires. However, through this book you can start to overcome your addiction. For example, it will help you take back control of your life and thus decrease your feelings of helplessness. You will be equipped with practical knowledge and theoretical knowledge that will help you feel more prepared, able, and motivated to combat your addiction. You will learn all about what addiction is and why you may be more at risk for addiction. You will even be led through several exercises to help curb your urges. Next, you will learn how to regulate your emotions and desires so that you're not so influenced by your addiction. No matter what your instinctive emotions are (whether you're alone or in company without access to your addiction), this book will teach you how to handle your emotions and control your subsequent actions. The important thing to note is that your emotions are not the enemy. It's okay to feel angry, frustrated, depressed, or anxious. You must accept these emotions, along with the reason for them, before you can effectively channel better emotions and actions. Another benefit you will gain from this book is that you will learn how to develop stronger and healthier relationships with others. Again, your addiction may have caused your relationships to suffer as you neglected your loved ones.

Alternatively, your addiction may be triggered by certain relationships wherein you're treated unfairly and unkindly. Either way, you will learn how to develop balanced relationships where you're neither taking advantage of others nor being taken advantage of by others. You will be led through how to form healthy, positive relationships.

There are countless benefits that you will gain from this book to help you overcome your addiction. To help you be more prepared and receptive to these benefits, here is an outline of what is to come so that you know what to expect. In Chapter 1, you will receive general information about addiction so that you understand your condition better. You will learn of the diagnostic criteria and symptoms of addiction. It's important to understand your condition so that you understand your own thoughts, emotions, and behaviors better. In Chapter 2, you will study the risk factors and negative effects associated with addiction. Understanding this will help you be kinder to yourself and prevent you from blaming yourself for your addiction. Such blame is unproductive and only serves to lower your self-perception, while simultaneously provoking your addiction. You will also be more determined to fight your addiction when you have a clear and undeniable view of how it is harming you.

In Chapter 3, you will begin learning the practical knowledge that will guide you to overcome your addiction. Specifically, you will receive cognitive behavioral therapy (CBT) exercises to increase your awareness of some faulty cognitions and replace them with more effective thought patterns. In Chapter 4, you will be led through some acceptance and commitment therapy (ACT) exercises. This form of treatment emphasizes embracing yourself and being dedicated to healing. In Chapter 5, you will learn how to conduct exposure and response prevention (ERP) therapy on yourself. This will help you confront the triggers of your addiction without succumbing to your urges. In Chapter 6, you will learn about relapses and how you must approach them. Relapses are to be expected when you're recovering from addiction. However, there are ways for you to recover from a relapse and prevent one too. You may not always be able to wholly prevent a relapse, though, so it's equally important to know how to recover from one. Finally, in Chapter 7, you will explore how to develop healthy relationships and how to incorporate your loved ones into your healing process. You will also discover how to give and receive forgiveness.

These are the categories of knowledge that you can expect to receive from this book. I truly believe that you will benefit and grow from the information provided to you here. In order to overcome addiction, I believe you need both practical and theoretical knowledge so that you can understand yourself better and practice the necessary habits that will combat your addiction. However, the most important part of your journey to recovery involves a simple choice: You must make the decision to start on this journey. All the information provided here will be useless if you don't decide to make full use of it. So, before you continue reading, renew the conviction in your heart to fight your addiction. This is the first step in defeating your addiction and taking back control of your life. So now, without further delay, let's start on the next step of your healing journey.

CHAPTER 1

What Is Addiction Anyway?

The best way to win in a fight is to understand your opponent. If you know how they fight, what tricks they might use against you, how they think, and so on, you will be in a better position to counter their moves and protect yourself. The same logic applies for the inner battle you're experiencing. You can't help yourself and fight your condition if you don't know what exactly it is you're fighting. So, the next step in your road to recovery is to fully understand what you're facing.

Explaining Addiction

Addiction can be understood as an inability to stop using a certain substance or engage in a certain behavior, despite knowing that it causes you psychological and or physical harm.

Linda Hill

Addiction is a chronic condition that can entail not being able to control your consumption of drugs (legal or illegal), as well as alcohol, foods, and so on. You will learn more about the different types of addiction later on. For now, let's continue defining what addiction is. Along with the definitions you've received so far, addiction can also be understood as a chronic (but treatable) medical disease that involves complex interactions between your brain circuits, genetics, life experiences, and environment. These interactions may make you more at risk of addiction, as they may make you more inclined to take part in compulsive behavior and more likely to continue abusing a substance despite the harmful consequences. Addiction can start from a place of curiosity, where you voluntarily start taking a substance (this is often, but not always, the case with addiction), or you may have been forced or peer pressured into trying a substance for the first time. Whether you voluntarily or involuntarily started taking a substance, addiction may have taken root in your mind and gradually lowered your self-control.

Coming from a biological view, addiction can be seen as a chronic dysfunction in your brain system involving reward, motivation, and memory. These systems will affect how your body craves a certain substance or behavior, how you weigh your desire for that substance or activity over the consequences

12

of it, and how you experience a compulsive or obsessive chase of the reward of engaging in your addiction. So, in terms of reward, your mind will zero in on those rewarding emotions associated with your addiction and you will feel intensely motivated to engage with it. You will feel strong urges and compulsions to indulge in your addiction. As for your memory, you may selectively choose to remember only the reward aspects of your past experiences with your addiction. This means that you will conveniently block out or disregard the real consequences you've experienced before in favor of the positive memories of your addiction. Therefore, you won't be overly concerned with the negative effects of your addiction. You will only be focused on getting the high or the reward associated with it.

As you've previously learned, addiction can be defined as a lack of control over your actions, where you may use or do something to the point that it's harmful to you. Common addictions are to drugs, smoking, alcohol, and gambling. However, addiction as a condition isn't limited to these substances. Addiction simply involves an inability to stop partaking in something. Therefore, it's possible to be addicted to anything. For example, you may be addicted to work, the internet, shopping, certain solvents, and so on. As long as you have the mindset of addiction, it can count as an addiction and you should take action against it. It may be hard for you to understand addiction outside the normal realms of drugs, alcohol, and the like, but addiction to other activities and substances are quite common and should be taken seriously. If you're addicted to work, you may be so obsessed with your performance and your status to the point where you work yourself to your physical limits. This may cause you to become physically exhausted, which will negatively affect your physical health. Socially, you will suffer, too, as you may neglect your family and friends. Rather than planning to spend any time with them, you may focus solely on your work, never taking holidays or even little breaks to call your loved ones.

If you're addicted to the internet, you may face the same issues. Your physical and social health may decrease as you spend more and more time alone and immobile. When you're glued to your phone or computer, you will stay in and be more inactive. This inactivity will negatively affect your physical health and you will gain weight easily. Being on your phone or laptop all day, even if you're using them to talk to others online, will still harm your social health, as you will become unfamiliar and uncomfortable with face-to-face interactions. This will lower your social skills. It may be hard to tell if you're addicted to the internet or not, especially since society today depends on the internet so heavily. A good indicator of internet addiction is if you spend hours every day and night using the internet while neglecting other important parts of your life. Another uncommon addiction that people may not be aware of is an addiction to shopping. This can also be a hard addiction to pinpoint, since online shopping is such a normal part of our lives now. It's convenient, and it can help you save money, so you may naturally start to shop more. On top of that, you may also go shopping at physical stores as a way to pass the time and socialize with your friends. These are all common and healthy reasons to shop. However, shopping may become an addiction when you start to buy things you don't need or want just to achieve a buzz. Often, this high may be followed by feelings of guilt, shame, or despair at having wasted your money on something that you don't need or want. This may then lead to more shopping in order to allay those negative feelings. This forms a vicious cycle of addiction and emotional distress.

As you can see, there are common and uncommon addictions. The more common addictions that are widely known are to alcohol, nicotine, marijuana, or pain relievers. Other common addictions that are less widely known (maybe because they pose less of an immediate threat to your physical health) are to coffee, gambling, food, technology, work, and sex. As with the examples provided above, it can be hard to tell when something is a healthy hobby or an addiction. Some habits or social behaviors may look like addiction when they're not. Other habits or social behaviors may look healthy, but they're actually signs of addiction. A good guideline for you to tell whether or not you're addicted is if you react negatively when you don't get access to your addiction or if you don't get your reward or high. For example, if you're addicted to coffee and you don't get it, you may experience some physical and psychological withdrawal symptoms such as fatigue, severe headaches, or irritability.

Diving deeper into common addictions, let's explore substance abuse or drug abuse. These terms entail a pattern of harmful uses of psychoactive substances, including all kinds of drugs (legal and illegal) and alcohol. These substances can lead you to be physically and psychologically dependent on them. When you're dealing with addiction, this is a word that you will hear a lot: dependent. What does this term mean? Dependence refers to a whole range of symptoms (physical, mental, and behavioral) that develop after you abuse a substance. Some key components of dependence are a strong craving to repeatedly and consistently abuse that substance, difficulties controlling your choice to abuse that substance or not, difficulties controlling how often you abuse that substance, and the persistent choice to abuse that substance despite its harmful effects on you. Drug abuse will inevitably harm your quality of life, as you will prioritize it over any other aspect of your life, thus leading you to neglect those parts and allowing them to deteriorate. For example, you will prioritize your addiction over any of your other social, interpersonal, educational, or occupational activities and responsibilities. Your sense of duty, obligation, or connection to others will be trumped by your compulsion and addiction. Other than lowering your emphasis on every other part of your life, drug abuse will intensify itself by increasing your tolerance of the substance. The more you take it, the higher your tolerance will become, and the more you will need of the substance the next time you take it in order to achieve the same effects and high.

There are a number of reasons why you may have started taking drugs. You may have been curious, you may have simply wanted to have some fun, or you may have seen others taking it and been pressured into it. Going on, you may have wanted to self-medicate in order to ease the effects or distract yourself from other problems. If you were going through a lot of stress or emotional distress, you may have turned to drugs to help you feel better. From there, you may have developed your addiction. One thing to note here is that drug use doesn't always result in dependence and addiction. There are certain risk factors (which you will study in the next chapter) that may influence how susceptible you are to addiction. However, a tell-tale sign that your drug use has become an addiction is when it begins to cause you problems in other spheres of your life, such as at home, at work, or at school. You will also notice that your social, physical, and mental health are being affected.

Now that you understand what addiction is, as well as the various types of addictions, let's briefly see what causes addictions. As you've read above, there may be various reasons why you first tried the substance that you're now addicted to. You may have been curious, you may have been pressured into it, and so on. But why did the addiction begin? You probably have many hobbies and have tried many things in your lifetime, and none of those things have developed into addictions. So, what makes this particular substance or activity so addictive? Well, if you're addicted to drugs, smoking, or nicotine, the answer is probably that these substances produce chemical changes in your body that affect how you feel physically and mentally. They produce enjoyable feelings in your brain and this creates a powerful compulsion to experience such feelings again. And in order to experience that pleasure and high again, you will feel strong urges to use those substances again. This starts you on the road to addiction. Other than substances, there are behavioral addictions where you're addicted to certain activities, such as gambling or shopping. These activities can create similar effects in your brain and lead you to achieve the same types of highs as the substances listed above. For example, when you win a round of poker or when you swipe your card on a purchase, you may feel elated and on top of the world. These positive emotions will be coupled with strong urges to recreate them, and this will lead you to compulsively and insistently engage in those activities.

It can be very difficult to stop engaging in these activities or substances, as your mind is intently fixed on the reward of engaging in them. If you don't, you may experience withdrawal symptoms as you come down from your high. These symptoms are intensely unpleasant, so in an effort to avoid those emotions and chase that high, you may continue indulging in your addiction, and this creates a cycle. To understand this cycle better, try to see addiction as a series of stages. As your brain and body progress along these stages, they will react and act differently. There are four main stages of addiction, and these are experimentation, social or regular, problem or risk, and dependency. In the beginning stages, you will start with experimentation, where you use a substance or engage in an activity simply out of curiosity. At this stage, you will enjoy the substance or activity, but you won't feel any intense urges to do them. Next is the social or regular stage, where you use or engage with the substance or activity for social reasons. This is a convenient excuse to start doing it regularly. At this point, you may start to feel some infrequent urges to do it. The third stage is the problem or risk stage, where you use or engage in the substance or activity in extreme ways. At this point, you will have little to no concern for the consequences of your actions. You will only focus on your intense urges and your desire to gain your rewards and highs. Lastly is the dependency stage, where you engage with your addiction on a daily basis, sometimes several times a day. You will also continue disregarding the negative consequences of your habits.

So far, you've received considerable information on what addiction is and how you can understand it. Equally important information to have, though, is what addiction isn't. This can help you differentiate between concepts and be confident about whether or not you're suffering from addiction. A common misconception that people confuse with addiction is misuse. Drug addiction and drug misuse are different concepts. Misuse suggests that you use a certain substance at overly high doses or in inappropriate situations that could result in health and social problems. Every drug comes with advice on its proper dose and how to use it. Drug misuse means that you ignore that advice and use it inappropriately. However, not everyone who misuses a drug is addicted to it. For example, if you drink a lot of alcohol on a night out and end up throwing up or blacking out, you can be said to be misusing a drug. However, unless you also experience compulsions to seek out that drug, and withdrawal symptoms when you don't have access to that drug, you can't be classified as having an addiction. So, you could understand drug misuse as applying to specific situations, while drug addiction applies to your overall lifestyle. Drug misuse is when you use substances in ways that you shouldn't, but usually you're able to stop if you want to. Addiction occurs when you can't stop. Even when it endangers your health, causes financial stress, increases emotional distress, and leads to problems in your interpersonal relationships, you won't be able to stop.

Symptoms of Addiction

Now that you understand what addiction is and isn't, let's become more aware of the signs and symptoms of addiction. Above, it was mentioned that it can be hard to tell when something progresses into addiction. Here, you will be taught all the various and extensive signs that can alert you to a possible addiction. According to the Diagnostic and Statistical Manual of Mental Disorders (DSM), substance use disorder (SUD) is defined as a pattern of symptoms caused by an individual using a substance continuously, despite the known negative effects it has on them. There are 11 basic criteria that can act as a guide to see if you have SUD. Of these 11 criteria, they all fall under four general categories: impaired control, social problems, physical dependence, and risky use. The criteria are:

- Using more of a substance than is advised or using a substance for longer than you're meant to

- Trying to decrease or stop using a substance, but not being able to

- Experiencing intense urges, cravings, and compulsions to use the substance

- Needing more and more of the substance to get the same desired effect (this is called tolerance)

- Developing withdrawal symptoms when you don't use the substance

- Spending more time acquiring and abusing drugs and substances

- Neglecting your obligations and responsibilities at home, work, or school due to your addiction

- Continuing to use the substance even though it causes problems in your relationships

- Giving up important and desirable social and recreational

activities that you used to enjoy due to substance abuse

- Using substances in settings that are risky and that put you in harm's way

- Continuing to use the substance regardless of the physical and mental health problems it causes you

These are the symptoms and signs that you have SUD. The number of these criteria that apply to you and the severity of the experience may differ. But as long as you suspect that you're addicted to something, you should reach out for help and take action to help yourself. If you're in the beginning stages of addiction, then these criteria may not affect you too strongly. But you should still take your condition seriously and do the necessary steps to heal yourself. In regard to the levels of severity for these symptoms, there are typically three levels of severity with addiction. Like any other sickness, it will worsen over time. Since it can be difficult to objectively quantify how much any one criteria affects you, you can measure the severity of your addiction by the number of criteria that apply to you. For example, if only one symptom applies to you, then you could be said to be at risk of SUD. If two or three criteria apply to you, it could point to a mild SUD. Four or five symptoms suggest moderate SUD. Six or more indicate severe SUD, which in turn suggests that you have an addiction to that substance.

Knowing how severe your symptoms are can help you figure out whether you're addicted, misusing, or at risk of misusing. This can help you plan the best course of action to take.

General signs of addiction are a lack of control, decreased socialization and increased isolation, and having a total lack of concern for your personal safety and health. The level of intensity at which you display these signs will increase as your addiction persists. A healthy person would be able to take note of their negative habits and work to get rid of them. However, if you have an addiction, you may choose to justify or ignore your behavior so that you can keep indulging in your addiction. Other behavioral signs of addiction are declining grades or difficulty at school, declining performance at work, relationship troubles, issues with employment, a lack of energy in daily activities, or changes in appearance. Addiction will significantly affect your behavior as you will have less control over yourself. All your attention and motivation will be geared toward your addiction. So, your grades or work performance will decline, as you won't be focused or motivated to do well. Your relationships will also suffer, as you won't prioritize your loved ones anymore. You may even experience a lack of energy when you're not indulging in your addiction, as you're now physically dependent on it to give you joy and energy. All these indicators can be a lot to remember so, as a helpful guide, an extensive but not exhaustive list of signs and symptoms of addiction can be seen below:

- Mood swings
- Anxiety
- Depression
- Irritability
- Euphoria
- Hyperactivity
- Agitation
- Decreased motivation
- Legal problems
- Unexplainable need for money
- Borrowing or stealing money from others
- Changes in friends, hangouts, and hobbies
- Loss of control over drug use
- Using the drug to relieve withdrawal symptoms
- Blackouts
- Drop in work or school attendance

- Deteriorating physical appearance
- Inattention to personal grooming habits
- Worsening of medical conditions
- Physical dependence
- Withdrawal effects if drug is discontinued
- Infections
- Changes in sleep or appetite
- Bloodshot eyes
- Pupils smaller or wider than usual
- Lethargy
- Decreased respiration rate
- Psychological dependence
- Worsening of mental illnesses
- Paranoia
- Hallucinations

- Changes in personality or attitude
- Fearfulness
- Aggressiveness
- Violent, angry outbursts

Those are the general signs that you are suffering from addiction. Now, let's discover in detail the symptoms of addiction in terms of your personality changes. After the experimentation stage of addiction, you may display some major or minor shifts in your behavior and personality. Such symptoms are listed above, such as a lack of interest in hobbies that used to be important to you, neglecting your interpersonal relationships, changes in your sleep patterns, increased alienation, and increased secrecy (about the amount of substance you use or the frequency at which you use it). One noticeable behavior change is that you will surround yourself with others who encourage your unhealthy habits. This way, you won't need to make excuses or justify your behavior to others. So, you may notice that you're spending time with a very different crowd.

Other signs show themselves through your mental and physical health. Some of these physical symptoms are listed above, such as having lower energy or bloodshot eyes. Other physical symptoms include constant sickness (such as flus or coughs), unexplained injuries, sudden changes in weight, bad skin, hair, teeth, and nails, along with sweating, trembling, vomiting, memory loss, and speech problems (such as slurred words or rambling). Similarly, some common mental symptoms were listed above, such as mood swings, irritability, and depression. Other than those, there are also apathy and suicidal thoughts. It's important to keep a close eye on these symptoms, as they can significantly harm your health. It's also important to recognize the full extent of your symptoms. Remember that people with addictions almost always underestimate the seriousness of their condition. This can cause them to ignore their symptoms, leading to long-term life consequences.

On a related note, there are also psychological symptoms of addiction. A common one that has been restated is an inability to stop using. This can come from a physiological cause (some substances are chemically addictive) or a psychological cause (where you've grown emotionally dependent on a substance in order to make you happy). Using a substance despite the harm it causes you can also be seen as a psychological symptom. This may initially come from a place of low self-worth and low self-esteem. You may be aware of the negative effects of a substance when you first start using it, but you may not care enough about yourself to stop. Moreover, another psychological symptom of addiction is obsession. You may become more and more obsessed with using a substance, gradually spending more time and energy to get it and use it. Next, taking risks is a sign of addiction, as you may incur high and unnecessary risks upon yourself in order to obtain the substance or engage in certain behaviors. Furthermore, you may engage in risky behaviors while under the influence of certain substances. For example, you may get into fights or drive recklessly. Taking an initial large dose is a common symptom of addiction, especially with alcohol. You may rapidly consume large amounts of a substance to quickly feel the effects and obtain a high.

From another angle, there are also social symptoms of addiction. Firstly, you have isolation, which can lead to solitude and secrecy. You also have sacrifices as a symptom, where you cross out other things in your life in order to fully focus on your addiction. This may be voluntary or involuntary. You may choose to forgo a camping trip with your friends because you won't have access to your addiction in the woods. Or you may be forced to stop playing your favorite sport because your physical health has been too affected by your addiction. Another social symptom of addiction is maintaining a good supply. Even if you're short on cash, you will find ways to ensure your supply of your addiction. You may even have little stashes hidden in different parts of your house or car to avoid detection. A very common social symptom is denial. You may not be aware of your addiction, or you may consciously try to deny it and refuse the need to seek help. You may lie to yourself, saying that you can quit whenever you want to. Having legal issues is a symptom listed above, but it wasn't explained then. This symptom simply refers to the common characteristic of people with alcohol and drug addictions. It also links back to the symptom of taking risks. When substances impair your judgment and increase your likelihood of taking risks, you may end up breaking the law or disrupting the public peace.

In this chapter, you've received extensive and in-depth explanations on what addiction is, and how to tell if you have one. This information will help you understand yourself and your condition better, and help you to confidently know whether or not you have an addiction. In the next chapter, you will learn about the risk factors and negative effects of addiction.

CHAPTER 2

The Befores and Afters of Addiction

In the previous chapter, you explored what to expect during your addiction. You learned what addiction is and the signs that alert you to an addiction. Now, let's discover the befores and afters of an addiction. That is, the risk factors that may have affected your development of an addiction, and the effects on your physical, mental, and social life once you've developed an addiction.

Risk Factors of Addiction

Risk factors are anything that may increase your risk of getting a certain disease or illness. For addiction, there are several that may have affected you. Keep in mind that there's a wide range of things that you may be addicted to, so this list may have a few factors that don't apply to you. Also, just because it's listed here doesn't mean that it automatically applies to you. You must reflect on yourself and your history to determine which risk factors may have played a role in your development of an addiction. This will help you understand yourself more and be kinder to yourself.

The first risk factor is genetics. This is a common risk factor that plays a significant role in addiction. Genetic vulnerability has been studied extensively in relation to addiction, and strong links have been verified, though the particular genes involved have not been isolated yet. The way your genes may make you more vulnerable to developing an addiction may have to do with your brain. When you abuse a substance or indulge in a particular activity (such as gambling, shopping, or using the internet), you activate certain reward pathways in your brain. This is more certain when you abuse a substance, as there are certain chemicals (such as dopaminergic neurons) that will definitely activate those areas. Anyway, these pathways are part of your survival instincts, as they will reward behaviors that are auspicious and helpful. For example, your reward pathways activate and you experience pleasure whenever you eat certain foods, such as those high in fat, salt, or sugar, which were vital for energy and survival as humans were evolving. Drugs and other possible activities bypass this behavior stage and stimulate your reward pathways directly, mimicking your happy hormones, such as endorphins. Where your genes play a role is that some people's reward pathways are more easily influenced or hijacked by drugs, while others are less easily influenced. This vulnerability is partly affected by your genes, which code for how sensitive your brain receptors are to drugs. There are several genes involved in this and you may have inherited a few through your parents or older generations.

The types of genes and degree of genetic vulnerability that factor into addiction vary for different drugs. For example, with tobacco, the genes that would make you more vulnerable to addiction are the ones involved in nicotine metabolism. For alcohol, it's the genes involved in alcohol metabolism and structuring certain brain cell receptors (such as the ones for serotonin or dopamine). For opioids, it's the genes that structure the brain cell receptors for opioids and the enzymes that metabolize opioids in your body. All these different genes affect your vulnerability to specific types of drugs. Other than that, many aspects of your drug use are influenced by your genetics. Your genes practically code for everything in your body, so they will also code for how your body interacts with a substance. For example, your genes may affect how pleasurable you find a drug, the quantity needed for an overdose, the long-term effects, the intensity of your withdrawal symptoms and cravings, and the rate at which you develop a tolerance. An easy way to see genetics playing a role in addiction is to observe the children of alcoholic fathers versus those of non-alcoholic fathers. The former group may tend to drink more, enjoy drinking more, and have better tolerance for alcohol.

Other than genetics, there are also personal factors that make you more vulnerable to addiction: personality traits. There are four main personality traits that may lead you to addiction: sensation-seeking, impulsiveness, anxiety sensitivity, and hopelessness. All these traits, except for sensation-seeking, are connected to mental health disorders, so they may concurrently make you more susceptible to addiction. If you're sensation-seeking, you may be drawn to abusing substances, as they can heighten your senses. If you're impulsive, you may fall into addiction, as you don't think before you act and continually chase that high. If you're sensitive to anxiety, you may experience a lot of emotional distress and rely on substances to allay those emotions. If you're prone to hopelessness, you may also rely on addiction to distract you or detract from that emotion.

On a related note, concurrent mental health disorders may increase your chances of developing an addiction. As mentioned above, the personality traits that are risk factors are linked to certain mental health disorders. So, if you have that disorder, you may also have that personality trait, which would make you more vulnerable to addiction. For example, if you have attention deficit and hyperactivity disorder or antisocial personality disorder, you may have the personality trait of impulsivity, which makes you vulnerable to addiction. In the modern day, many people suffer from a variety of mental health issues, many of which are linked to a higher risk of developing an addiction. Each mental health disorder has different traits and habits that may put you at risk of addiction. Borderline personality disorder involves a pattern of unstable interpersonal relationships, low self-image, volatile emotions, and high impulsivity. Antisocial personality disorder is associated with egocentric identity, pleasure-seeking habits, and a lack of empathy for others. These are all traits and mental health disorders that may increase your risk of addiction. Other mental health disorders such as depression, anxiety, post-traumatic stress disorder, schizophrenia, and other psychotic illnesses also increase your chances of addiction, as you may self-medicate using substances or other activities. In an effort to treat your symptoms and alleviate your emotional distress, you may indulge in drugs, gambling, or other activities. This may be effective in the short-term, but over time your tolerance will grow, and you will need more and more of the substance to feel okay.

Though there is a clear correlation between mental health

disorders and addiction, there is no firm causation that has been established yet. Having a mental health disorder may make you more vulnerable to addiction. Having an addiction may also make you more vulnerable to developing a mental health disorder. The one type of addiction that has been studied more extensively on this topic is alcohol. People who abuse alcohol are more at risk for mood disorders, such as depression, while people with mood disorders are more likely to abuse alcohol to cope with their symptoms. This is because alcohol can create an organic mood syndrome that is clinically impossible to distinguish from a primary mood disorder. And alcohol may temporarily relieve the symptoms of someone with a mood disorder, but in the long run, it can significantly worsen their mood. In fact, all major drugs can worsen your mood in the long run, which is why addiction is closely related to mental health disorders.

Going back to your developmental stages, there are several developmental factors that may increase your risk of addiction. The first risk factor is early use. If you began using a substance in your adolescence, you're more likely to have developed a problematic relationship with that substance as you grew up. Using substances in your adolescence can result in potentially lifelong ramifications, as it interferes with your brain development and social transitions. The next risk factor is your family. Your relationship with your parents actually plays a big role in your vulnerability to addiction. For example, parental monitoring, open communication, supervision, and close relationships between parents and children can deter the child's involvement in risky behavior. Authoritative parenting usually leads to the best outcome for teens. This is in contrast to authoritarian or permissive parenting. Authoritative parenting is when there's a firm hand and clear rules for the child, but still room for them to explore, grow, and make mistakes. Authoritarian parenting is when there's absolute control over the child and no room for them to explore, grow, and make mistakes (this can make them rebellious, suppressed, resentful, ignorant, easily manipulated, and so on). Permissive parenting is when there's no control at all over the child, and so they're left to do whatever they want with no consequences, values, or rules to follow (this is dangerous, as they have no idea as to what's right or wrong). Moving on, children may be less likely to use substances if their parents talked more openly about substance use to them. Contrastingly, children may be more likely to use substances if they see their parents using them too.

Continuing on the risk factor of family, siblings play a role as well. If an older sibling uses a substance during adolescence and early adulthood, a younger sibling may be more likely to use that substance too. However, the strength of this influence is affected by the quality of the sibling relationship. If there is a warm, close, and supportive relationship, the younger sibling is more likely to model themselves after the older sibling. This is particularly true if the siblings are of the same gender and age. Other aspects of your family that may affect your risk of addiction is family conflict and disharmony, family disorganization (having a lack of stability), and low family cohesion (having a lack of connectedness, bonds, or involvement with family members).

Another developmental factor that's a risk factor is trauma. If you experienced early childhood trauma, you're more susceptible to drug misuse. The more stress you were exposed to as a child, the higher your chances of becoming addicted to substances. If you were abused (emotionally, physically, or sexually), neglected, witnessed domestic violence, lost a parent by death or divorce, witnessed a parent with addiction or other mental health disorders, or had a parent who was incarcerated, you are much more likely to develop an addiction compared to people who didn't experience these things as children. Childhood trauma isn't the only kind of trauma that increases your risk of addiction. Trauma experienced later in life can cause you to develop post-traumatic stress disorder which, as mentioned before, can be a risk factor for addiction.

Moreover, your peers are a developmental factor that can

increase your risk of addiction. Your peers may play a vital role in your use of substances by providing consensual validation for those experiences. Especially in your adolescence, you trust your peers the most, as you feel closest to them. They provide you with a break from the adult worlds of school and home, help you build your identity, offer opportunities for romantic relationships, and fuel your sensation-seeking and risky behaviors. Your peers are typically the ones who initiate and escalate your use of alcohol, tobacco, and certain illicit drugs. The last developmental factor is spirituality. Having high levels of spirituality and religiosity may reduce your risk of addiction and substance abuse, both as an adolescent and as an adult.

Social factors are another category of risk factors that increase your chances of addiction. Social isolation is a big factor that may cause you to measure risk and reward differently compared to the brain of someone more social. This makes a socially isolated person more sensitive toward the reward of drugs. Your lack of social connections may make you crave drugs more intensely, as they both activate the same pathways in your brain. By abusing certain substances, you can achieve the same neurobiological sensations of social connection. Negative socialization (such as being bullied or peer pressured) is also a major risk factor.

So far, the risk factors have all had to do with you—your family, your genetics, your personality traits, and so on. But there are also external risk factors that most people don't consider, which are the drug characteristics. How easily you may get addicted to a certain drug varies from substance to substance. There are various critical factors of a drug that affect your development of drug dependence. The main five are:

- Withdrawal: Some drugs don't produce withdrawal symptoms while others do. Of this latter category, some drugs produce severe symptoms, while others produce mild ones.

- Reinforcement: This is the measure of a substance's ability to get you to take it repeatedly, and as a replacement to other substances.

- Tolerance: This is a measure of how much of the substance is needed to satisfy your (often increasing) cravings for it.

- Dependence: This factor relates to how hard it is for you to stop using this substance, the relapse rate, the percentage of users who become dependent, the ratings users give to their own need for the substance, and the degree to which the substance will continue being used in the face of hard evidence that it's causing harm to the user.

- Intoxication: The level of intoxication caused by a substance may increase the level of pleasure you feel (while also increasing the potential personal and social damage it may cause).

Other than these factors, there's also the route of administration which affects how quickly a drug works. The faster it reaches your brain, the higher your risk of addiction. The fastest routes of administration are injection, smoking, snorting, and swallowing, in that order. Certain drugs reach your brain very quickly and give you a short but intense high. These drugs are highly addictive.

The last factor to touch on is the severity of your withdrawal symptoms. This was briefly mentioned above, but deserves deeper consideration. Withdrawal symptoms can lead to addiction simply because you keep using the substance to avoid the severe side effects you suffer from when you stop. Prolonged drug use can increase the severity of your withdrawal symptoms, as it can lead to tolerance, which is a sign of physical dependency on a substance. It's important to state that physical dependency and addiction aren't the same thing. Addiction differs in that it has a psychological component, as well, that leads to cravings and compulsions to use a drug, even without withdrawal symptoms. Nevertheless, drugs that produce severe withdrawal symptoms can be the most addictive, as these symptoms reinforce your consumption of the drug. Drugs that quickly leave your bloodstream (such as cocaine) can produce withdrawal symptoms within hours, leaving you craving the drug. Some of the most addictive substances are nicotine, heroine, cocaine, alcohol, and meth. These substances have severe withdrawal symptoms and can result in quickly-developed tolerance.

Effects of Addiction

The risk factors of addiction cover the befores of developing an addiction. There are various factors that may apply to you that enhance your susceptibility to addiction. Next are the effects of addiction, which can span across your physical, mental, and social state. Physically, you may experience changes in coordination, blood pressure, and heart rate, being either more awake or more sleepy, improved sociability, pain relief, and changes in appearance. These are the short-term effects. Long-term effects will begin after a prolonged period of abuse. Moreover, the specific physical effects of drugs vary based on the individual, the substance, the dosage, the delivery method, and the duration of use. The following are examples of common drugs that people become addicted to, along with their short-term physical effects:

- Alcohol: impaired coordination, raised heartbeat, reddening of skin, rashes, dizziness, vomiting, nausea, potential coma, increased physical activity, decreased appetite, irregular heart rate, increased blood pressure and temperature.

- Cocaine: narrowed blood vessels, higher body temperature, heart rate, and blood pressure, enlarged pupils, headaches, nausea, heart attack, stroke, seizure, coma, abdominal pain, erratic and violent behavior.

- Benzodiazepines: slurred speech, lower coordination, lower blood pressure, dizziness, slower breathing.

- Heroin and opioids: dry mouth, nausea, vomiting, slower breathing, slower heart rate.

- Tobacco and nicotine: higher blood pressure, heart rate, and breathing, greater risk of lung cancer (due to smoking).

And these are the long-term physical effects (which are dependent on the type of substance, amount you consume, and how long you've been consuming it):

- Alcohol: heart disease, stroke, liver disease, liver inflammation, pancreatitis, cancer (breast, throat, mouth, voice box, liver, rectum, colon), digestive problems, and weakened immune system.

- Methamphetamines: dental problems, intense itching, weight loss, and other diseases from sharing needles.

- Cocaine and heroin: loss of your sense of smell, nasal damage, trouble swallowing, infection and death of bowel tissue from decreased blood flow, weight loss, collapsed veins, constipation, stomach cramps, liver or kidney disease, and infection of the lining and valves of the heart.

- Tobacco and nicotine: greatly increased risk of cancer (due to smoking), bronchitis, and heart disease.

As you can see, the physical effects of drugs and addiction can be far-reaching and impact almost every organ in your body. In general, this will lead to a weakened immune system, increased vulnerability to illnesses and infections, heart conditions (such as abnormal heart rates, collapsed veins, or heart attacks), liver damage, brain damage, problems with memory, attention, and decision-making, and even death.

However, just reading that addiction can adversely affect you in this way may not be convicting or convincing enough. So, let's study in detail how substance abuse can harm you on a biological level. In terms of your respiratory system, smoking cigarettes, cocaine, or marijuana may cause you to develop several issues and chronic pulmonary diseases such as chronic bronchitis, lung cancer, or emphysema. Significant respiratory depression can be caused by several substances, such as opioids and central nervous system depressants (sedatives, alcohol, and benzodiazepines). In severe cases, this respiratory depression can be fatal, and the risk is further heightened if you combine these drugs. Other respiratory complications include injury to your upper airway (caused by sniffing drugs), collapsed lungs (caused by inhaling drugs), community-acquired pneumonia (caused by injecting drugs), fatal asthma attacks, interstitial lung disease, pulmonary edema or vascular disease, septic embolism, and lung inflammation or infection (caused by foreign particulates that are found in many prescription and illegal drugs).

Your cardiovascular system is also affected by your addiction. As mentioned above, drugs can cause irregular heart rates and even heart attacks. The altered heart rate, heart rhythms, and blood pressure caused by drugs all increase your risk of cardiovascular issues, such as strokes or myocardial infarctions.

Next is your liver—the primary site of metabolism where most drugs pass through. This function of the liver makes it particularly susceptible to injury, as the more drugs you abuse, the harder your liver must work. Alcohol in particular has an adverse effect on your liver. Almost half of all deaths that were caused by liver disease were alcohol related. It's a commonly known fact that drinking too much can damage your liver. A lesser known fact is that acetaminophen is also toxic to your liver if taken excessively or over the prescribed doses. This drug can cause fulminant hepatic necrosis, or acute liver failure. Many opioid painkillers contain acetaminophen, so you may not even be aware that you're consuming it. But if you're addicted to such opioids or painkillers, it may result in serious liver injury. Also, injecting drugs into your system may increase your risk of contracting hepatitis B and C, which may lead to cirrhosis of the liver and liver cancer.

Another important organ in your body that suffers due to drug addiction is your kidneys. Every drug you take will ultimately pass through your kidneys before being excreted through your urine. High alcohol consumption can lead to a severe decline in renal function and increase your risk of chronic kidney disease. Illicit drugs also harm your kidneys, as they cause your body to dehydrate, heat up, and break down its muscles. Cocaine and heroin in particular are linked with acute glomerulonephritis, nephrotic syndrome, and interstitial nephritis (basically a cluster of symptoms such as fatigue, higher levels of urinary protein, and severe edema).

Entire systems in your body are even impacted by addiction. For example, your gastrointestinal system—as seen through the symptoms of nausea, vomiting, constipation, and diarrhea that are linked to several substances and their withdrawal symptoms. For instance, using opioids may cause you severe constipation, whereas its withdrawal symptoms include diarrhea. Other harms include acid reflux (from using opioids), and abdominal pain, bowel tissue decay, and mesenteric ischemia (from using cocaine). Being addicted to alcohol can lead to gastric, duodenal ulcers, gastrointestinal bleeding, esophageal cancer, and esophagitis.

Your brain is another organ in your body, and an important one at that, which is harmed by your addiction. Some of these harms are reversible, while others aren't. For example, using marijuana consistently in adolescence is linked with neuropsychological decline that doesn't seem to fully reverse even after halting use. Meanwhile, alcohol abuse is associated with various types of abnormal brain structure (such as impairment of white matter microstructure) and cognitive decline. If you're an alcoholic, you have a higher risk of developing dementia later in life and suffering from widespread brain atrophy. Other than these specific cases, substance abuse changes the way your brain responds to rewards. This means that, over time, the natural and healthy activities that you used to enjoy will lose their appeal and no longer provide you with satisfying or rewarding feelings. This will leave you more heavily reliant on the drug to give you the desired level of pleasure. And the amount of the substance needed to feel the same reward will continue increasing. Consequently, you may start to feel unmotivated, depressed, hopeless, and detached from past activities that you used to enjoy.

The brain chemical that is highly linked to how your brain responds to rewards is dopamine. This chemical regulares your emotions and feelings of pleasure. When you use certain substances, they may cause dopamine to flood your brain, creating a high. The pursuit of this high is one of the main causes of addiction. As you continue using a substance, it may alter your brain chemistry and change how your brain performs or makes choices. That is, you may start to feel intense cravings and prioritize getting that high over any other considerations (such as safety or responsibilities).

Other than the physical effects of addiction, there are also mental effects such as cognitive and behavioral changes. One reason for this is that addiction can exacerbate the symptoms of other mental disorders. For example, frequent cannabis use during adolescence can increase your risk of psychosis in adulthood. Other factors that impact how a substance affects your mental state include the type of substance and the frequency at which you take it. The short-term mental effects of addiction based on the substance you're using are as follows:

- Alcohol: euphoria, reduced anxiety, increased confidence, easier social interactions, and irritability and anxiety upon withdrawal.

- Cannabis: enhanced sensory perceptions, lower concentration, euphoria, relaxation, paranoia, and anxiety and irritability upon withdrawal.

- Benzodiazepines: difficulty concentrating, drowsiness, dizziness, reduced anxiety, and trouble remembering things.

- Heroin: euphoria, and restlessness upon withdrawal.

- Opioids: pain relief, euphoria, and drowsiness.

- Methamphetamine: increased alertness, and anxiety upon withdrawal.

And the long-term effects of addiction to these substances are:

- Alcohol: depression, social problems, anxiety, learning and memory problems.

- Opioids: increased risk of overdose.

- Methamphetamines: confusion, anxiety, insomnia, violent behavior, mood swings, delusions, paranoia, and hallucinations.

- Heroin: increased risk of overdose.

- Tobacco and nicotine: attention issues, sleep issues, depression upon withdrawal, attention and learning issues (especially if taken in adolescence), and irritability.

- Cannabis: mental health problems, insomnia, anxiety, and irritability upon withdrawal.

Other general short-term and long-term behavioral problems that may arise from addiction are aggression, impaired judgment, impulsiveness, and loss of self-control. These traits can cause you to lose your job, get into accidents, commit punishable offenses, and injure yourself. You may get involved in domestic violence, driving while intoxicated, or property damage cases. When you're addicted to something, your self-control goes out the window and you may impulsively do things you wouldn't normally.

The final area of your life that's affected by your addiction is your social life. In terms of your relationships or your marriage, your addiction can cause unspeakable grief for your other half. You may have changed significantly due to your addiction, becoming someone who is prone to mood swings, secrecy, aggression, violence, and other extreme behaviors. This can be hard for your partner or your friends to navigate and moderate, and it's even worse if you have children. For children, it can be confusing and distressing to see a parent exhibit signs of addiction. The children won't understand what's happening, and this will only make the whole experience scarier for them. Something that adds to the relationship strain is that you may be suffering from financial difficulties that your loved ones aren't aware of. This may cause you significant amounts of stress. Combined with the irrational actions, paranoia, secrecy, and volatile habits of your addiction, you may be heading for a full relationship breakdown. If you're addicted to something and desperate for your next hit, you may resort to violence and aggression to get what you want. You may threaten your partner or exploit them for money. The sad truth is that you'll put your cravings for your addiction far ahead of anything else, including your partner's safety and happiness. You will be solely motivated by your addiction. This can make you selfish, unempathetic, self-centered, and oblivious to their needs and concerns.

Your family will also be affected by your addiction, as they may feel helpless to guide you in overcoming it. They may be unsure of what course of action to take, and inadvertently take the wrong one in an effort to help you. This is often the case, as people desperately want to help, but don't know how. In the end, they may hurt you more than help you. For example, they may try to shame you into quitting, ostracize you until you get better, or deny that you have a problem. Sometimes, they may choose the worst possible ways to try to help you. But it's important to remember that their intentions are loving and caring.

Other than relationships, your education will be harmed as well. If you're addicted to a substance or activity, a common result is being truant from school. You may also start to exhibit antisocial behavior, such as stealing (to fund your addiction) or violent behavior (as a result of the impulsiveness or irritability of your addiction). Your grades will also drop, as you will have impaired concentration and low motivation. The substance you're using may harm your concentration, while your cravings for it will harm your motivation to pursue anything else. Rather than studying, you will spend large amounts of time thinking and planning how to get more of your addictive substance or activity.

In the same way, your employment will be affected by an addiction. Where you used to be smart, punctual, and efficient, you may suddenly transform into someone who is constantly tardy, unmotivated, neglectful of their appearance, and may

Linda Hill

display unacceptable and erratic behavior. You may shrug off certain duties (due to a lack of motivation), start stealing from your company (to fund your addiction), or consistently miss work (because you're hungover or facing withdrawal symptoms). This may cause you to lose your job, which in turn will further harm your family and relationships. Losing your job means you'll have no income, and this can put a strain on your romantic relationships.

Your personality will also undergo drastic changes which will affect your social relationships. However, how your addiction affects your personality is impacted by your psychological make up before the addiction, including your lifestyle and physical health. The substance you're using plays a role, too, as certain substances (such as heroin) have stronger effects upon your mental health and brain than other substances (such as nicotine). When your addiction starts to harm your personality, your peers, loved ones, and colleagues may notice these changes fairly quickly. You will begin to act totally out of character. For example, you may become secretive, offensive, deceitful, calculative, paranoid, restless, untrusting, having low self-esteem, arrogant, uncaring, and selfish. Your actions may also become alarming, displaying acts such as self-harm, stealing, or cutting off old friends and spending more time with people you don't know.

As mentioned previously, issues with the law are a common effect of addiction. This is because you will have lower impulse control, higher risk-taking habits, and low concern for the consequences of your actions. When added together, these traits allow addicts to often turn to crime as a way to pay for their addiction. Other run-ins with the law may include the rowdiness and drunkenness that comes with whatever substance you're using. For example, when you drink too much, you may become more aggressive and destructive. If this spills over into destruction of property or disruption of the public peace, then you may need to answer to the law. These are the various negative effects of addiction. Obviously, the effects are many and pervasive, affecting every part of your life and significantly lowering your quality of life. Knowing these effects in detail should encourage you to be more determined and motivated to overcome your addiction. With that said, the next chapter starts you on the practical exercises and therapies you can conduct on yourself in order to combat your addiction.

CHAPTER 3

Cognitive Behavioral Therapy

In this chapter, you will learn about cognitive behavioral therapy (CBT), how it works, and the specific practices you can do to help overcome your addiction. CBT is a kind of psychotherapeutic treatment that can help you discover how to identify and change your disturbing, distressing, and destructive thought patterns that have a negative impact on your actions and emotions. You may have several automatic negative thoughts that provoke and worsen your emotional distress and addictive habits. CBT aims to make you more aware of these thoughts and help you to change them. You will identify, challenge, and replace such thoughts with ones that are more objective, realistic, and helpful. This one branch of therapy encompasses several other types of techniques and approaches that focus on your thoughts, actions, and emotions. These therapeutic approaches are:

- Cognitive therapy: This treatment method focuses on identifying your inaccurate or distorted thought patterns, emotional responses, and actions. Once you've identified these thoughts, you can begin to change and redirect them.

- Dialectical behavior therapy: This focuses on your thoughts and behaviors, and aims to equip you with strategies that can regulate your emotions, such as mindfulness.

- Multimodal therapy: This treatment method posits that your psychological issues are best treated by addressing seven distinct but interconnected modalities. These seven modalities are your behavior, affect, sensation, cognition, imagery, interpersonal factors, and drug or biological factors.

- Rational emotive behavior therapy: This treatment assumes that your emotional distress is caused by your irrational beliefs. As such, it focuses on identifying these beliefs, actively challenging them, and learning to recognize and redirect these erroneous thought patterns.

All these subcategories of CBT adopt different approaches, but they all fundamentally aim to address your underlying thought patterns that may be provoking your psychological and emotional distress.

There are various techniques of CBT that function to accomplish this aim. The first technique is identifying negative thoughts. Your thoughts have a powerful impact on your emotions and actions, so it's important to learn how your thoughts, feelings, and circumstances can contribute to your addiction or other maladaptive habits. This technique requires a lot of introspection, which may be very tiring and uncomfortable, but at the end of the day, you will be led to new insights about yourself and many self-discoveries that may be vital to your healing process. Another CBT technique is practicing new skills. Your addiction, or any other psychological disorder, may be provoked or worsened by your maladaptive coping skills and other negative habits. So, CBT tries to treat your addiction or disorder by teaching you new skills that you can use in your life. Once you learn better coping skills and healthier reactions, you can prevent your condition from worsening and facilitate your healing.

Goal setting is also a CBT technique that can improve your overall quality of life. As you strive to improve your mental health, you will need to make some changes to improve your life and your health. This can be difficult to achieve if you don't know how to make and plan achievable and sustainable goals.

So, a common CBT technique, that a therapist may impart to you, is how to identify your goals, categorize them into short or long-term goals, make your goals SMART (specific, measurable, attainable, relevant, and time-based), and emphasize the journey as much as the destination. Moving on, problem-solving skills are a CBT technique that can sustain your progress and prevent potential relapses. When you know how to problem solve, you will be able to identify and adeptly overcome any problems that come from the stressors in your life. This will then reduce the negative reactions and impacts you face from your psychological illness. With CBT, problem solving involves five steps: identify the problem, make a list of possible solutions, evaluate the strengths and weaknesses of those solutions, choose the best solution to implement, and implement the solution. Finally, another well-known technique with CBT is self-monitoring. This is where you track your behaviors, symptoms, and experiences over time and reflect on them. You can do this by keeping a diary or making a note on your phone whenever something notable happens to you. For example, for people facing addiction, self-monitoring may involve keeping track of how often you feel your cravings and what triggered them.

CBT is a highly effective treatment method that can help you focus on your present and overcome your thinking errors.

Other than addiction, CBT is also helpful with anxiety, depression, eating disorders, personality disorders, bipolar disorder, anger issues, and phobias. It can also be used to help treat people experiencing serious physical illnesses, divorce, grief, low self-esteem, insomnia, relationships problems, and poor stress management. CBT is helpful for a wide range of experiences, as it can bring about several benefits. For example, it can help you engage in healthier thinking patterns. By making you more aware of your negative and unrealistic thinking patterns, you will become more conscious of how your thoughts can dampen your feelings and moods. This awareness will allow you to challenge your negative thoughts and make a conscious choice to engage in healthier and more positive thinking patterns. CBT is also an effective short-term treatment option. If you're facing a short-term problem, such as relationship problems or grief (as opposed to long-term problems that can affect your personality and every part of your life, such as addiction, depression, and other psychological disorders), then CBT can be very useful to you. Improvements can usually be seen within five to 20 sessions. This efficacy is still true whether the therapy is administered online or face-to-face. This is a huge benefit as many things have gone online now. Having access to online therapy can make it more convenient and flexible for the patient, thus increasing the probability that they'll return for more sessions. And one of the greatest benefits of CBT is that it equips you with helpful coping skills that are useful now, as you're fighting your psychological battle, and in the future, as you're sustaining your progress and dealing with the inevitable highs and lows of life. The skills you learn through CBT will not only help you overcome your addiction, they are even applicable in everyday life.

Despite all these benefits, there are a few things to consider, as well as challenges to expect while you're embarking on CBT treatment. The first is simply that change can be difficult. The root problem that you're dealing with in CBT is your automatic negative thoughts or reactions that you've probably had for years. Such habits can be deeply solidified in your mind. So, while you may become more aware of your thoughts which aren't healthy or rational, simply recognizing these thoughts may not make it easy for you to alter them. With that being said, remember to keep challenging yourself to change. And be patient with yourself—don't expect yourself to completely and immediately eradicate the thoughts and reactions you've had for so long. Another challenge of CBT is that it's very structured. This may not be a burden to you if you're naturally a structured and focused person. But if you're not, then CBT may cause a bit of discomfort for you. CBT doesn't usually focus on underlying unconscious resistances to treatment. Rather, it focuses more on psychoanalytic psychotherapy. This will be most effective for you if you're comfortable being instructed a lot and following directions.

On a related note, you as a patient must be willing to change. In order for CBT to be effective, you must be willing to listen to your therapist, spend time and energy analyzing your thoughts, confront things about yourself that may cause you distress or discomfort, and spend the necessary time and energy to change your behaviors and thoughts. The overall process of CBT can be arduous and tiring, but it's a great way to learn more about yourself and become more conscious of how you think. Finally, CBT can be challenging, as the progress is usually gradual. You won't suddenly wake up one day and be all better. CBT will help you take small, incremental steps toward changing your behavior and improving your mental health. You will slowly overcome your addiction—so slowly that you may not notice the improvements at first. You may start to experience fewer cravings or simply be more capable of handling your cravings. Or maybe you will be more capable of confronting your triggers and resisting your habits of addiction. Step-by-step, CBT will help you work toward the larger goal of overcoming your addiction and achieving holistic health. Anyway, these are the potential challenges that you may experience as you learn the skills of CBT. But knowing these in advance can help you predict, circumvent, and persevere through whatever challenges may come your way. So, without further delay, let's learn your first CBT skill.

SMART Goal Setting

Whenever you set out to achieve something (whether that's finishing a book, improving your grades, or overcoming your addiction), you set a goal for yourself. The success rate of you achieving that goal relies heavily on how you go about setting this goal. This exercise will bring you through how to set goals that increase your chances for success. The first step to this exercise is to set aside around 30 minutes for yourself to reflect on what your aims are and to define your intentions. As you're reflecting, write down your goals. Once you've done that, take a look at each goal and make sure that they are SMART (specific, measurable, attainable, relevant, and time-bound). For 'S,' you must make your goal specific. Write down your objective as an instruction where you tell yourself what to do. In other words, write it down as a specific statement. If your goal is vague, then your conviction, motivation, and plans of action will be vague as well. If you write down your goal as "I want to improve my studies," you may be lost as to how exactly you can achieve this goal. Instead, you should write down your goals so as to include the method rather than the outcome. For example, if you write "I want to increase my weekly study time by studying science for half an hour after dinner three times a week," then you will have an objective to work toward (improving your grades in science) and a clear plan on how to do so. By making a specific and activity-related goal, you define your aims and pathways more clearly.

One tip for making your goals as specific as possible is to try to make more "approach goals" rather than "avoidance goals." Approach goals (where you set a goal for an action that you want to take) are more effective than avoidance goals (where you set a goal for an action that you want to avoid). Moreover, "mastery goals" may be more effective than "performance goals." Performance goals are goals that aim to achieve a specific outcome. For example, "I want to get an A in math" or "I want to lose 15 pounds." Mastery goals are goals that focus on learning a new skill or increasing your pre-existing skills. Mastery goals may be more effective than performance goals, as the mindset that they encourage are different. Performance goals highlight your final performance and place little emphasis on your efforts and journey. All that matters is your final isolated performance. This isn't an objective or fair way to assess yourself. Meanwhile, mastery goals highlight your overall progress and efforts. That way, if any challenges arise, you can view them not as a hamper to your final performance, but as a natural part of chasing your goals. This encourages an active engagement in your goal-achievement process and increases your problem-solving skills. For example, if your goal is to practice a certain skill for a specific amount of time every day and certain circumstances arise to prevent you from meeting that goal, you may need to adapt and improvise to meet your goal. In contrast, challenges that arise as you're chasing a performance goal are often interpreted as failures of your abilities. This may lead you to feelings of defeat and frustration.

For the 'M' part of SMART goals, make your goals measurable by adding quantifiable criteria. This will help you measure your progress. If your goal isn't measurable, you will have a hard time deciding when enough is enough, when you can feel good about your progress, or when you can give yourself a break. On the flip side, making your goals measurable can help you feel good about your definite progress (it always feels good to be able to count off the numbers as you progress) and prevent you from underworking or overworking yourself. This will keep you motivated to keep progressing and create a sustainable process where you don't tire yourself out. Measuring your results can even help you adjust your goals as you go along. If you feel like you can do more or like you're doing too much and burning yourself out, adjust your measurements accordingly to make sure you can keep working at this goal in the long run. Some tips on making your goals measurable are to consider creative methods of tracking your progress. There may not always be easily measurable tools to track your progress, but don't let this deter you. Improvise something fun and creative to keep track of your progress. Another tip is, if you want to reduce stress, try to take some meditation breaks every day. It can be tiring and stressful to keep pursuing your goals, so give yourself a break and some time to relax. Keep track of these meditation breaks so that you can notice any trends or situations that spike your stress. Once you're aware of these trends, you can avoid them or respond more effectively in the future.

The 'A' in SMART stands for attainable. If you set large, looming goals that seem impossible to achieve, you may lose motivation and never start working toward those goals at all. To make your goals more attainable, break them into smaller goals and be specific and detailed about how you will achieve them. Your goals should be ambitious and possible. If you create goals for yourself that are hard to do or unhealthy to achieve (such as pushing yourself to lose 20 pounds in two weeks), you will lose confidence in yourself and motivation to change. This will cause you to become complacent about your condition and inactive in your own life. Instead, choose goals that will challenge you, but that you're confident you can reach through hard work. Making your goals attainable requires a lot of reflection, as you must ensure that you're not being too hard on yourself, not going too easy on yourself, being totally realistic about the work you'll need to put in, and being rational about the individual steps you've planned. Once you've ensured all of this, your goals will be attainable, and this will significantly increase your chances of success. An important thing to remember is that you can always make adjustments to your goals. What was attainable in the past may now be either too easy or too hard. Circumstances also change, and you may no longer have the time, supplies, or location in which to realistically meet your goals. When these things happen, remember to be flexible, and to make the proper alterations to your methods and goals.

Next, the 'R' in SMART stands for relevant. This means that your goals should be of some personal importance to you and that each step of attaining your goal should make sense to you. If you set a goal that's not really important or relevant to you (for example, if you're only doing it for someone else), then you may not feel motivated or dedicated to achieve your goal. Your goals should be yours—they should come from a place of personal importance, relevance, passion, or interest. All these will increase your conviction and increase your chances of success. One thing to note here is that sometimes you may have a goal that goes against some of your emotions, but this is still a worthy goal if it's in your best interest. For example, you may aim to increase your physical activity, and this goal may be protested against by your inner laziness or spirit of procrastination. But as long as you can recognize that it's good for you, then it may be a worthy goal. This higher purpose of improving your health and quality of life should be inspiring enough that it motivates you to succeed or at least to keep trying. For other goals where you're doing it for others and can't see the benefit you're getting from it, you probably won't be very determined to meet those goals. Obstacles on those paths will be very difficult to overcome and you will be less likely to work toward those goals. This is why others can keep advising you on what you should do to take care of yourself, but if you're not inspired by those statements and advice, you won't make any changes. You need to realize for yourself the legitimacy of a certain goal in order for it to become relevant to you. Only the goals you set for yourself will be meaningful to you, and those are the goals that you will be willing to put in the work for.

Finally, the 'T' in SMART means time-bound. This relates to when you predict you will achieve your goal. This prediction can't be too soon (as you must give yourself a realistic time period in which to achieve your goals) or too far off in the future (as this may make you lose motivation). By making your goals time-bound, you can provide yourself with a reasonable schedule and a foreseeable finish line that will motivate you to work toward it. For example, "I will get stronger this year" sets a vague timeline that is far in the future. This will allow you to procrastinate, thinking that you have all year to work on this goal. However, "I will exercise for an hour three times a week for three months" provides a specific, time-bound goal that you can measure, and a finish line that is far enough in the future for you to see progress, but not so far in the future that you can procrastinate. Once you reach the end of those three months, you can evaluate your progress and set new goals based on your current condition. These are the five criteria for making your goals SMART. As you're doing this exercise, read through the explanations for each criteria a few times and make sure you're following them.

You can use this template as you do this exercise to set your SMART goals: "I aim to (insert your goal here) by (insert how you will achieve this goal). I will know that I'm making progress on this goal because (insert how you will measure the goal) for (insert the time period for your goal)." An example of how to use this template is: "I aim to increase my physical strength by doing weight training at the gym three times a week for the next three months. I will know that I'm making progress on this goal because I will track the weights I'm lifting in a workout log every week for three months."

This exercise has led you through how you can set better goals for yourself. Now, here are some tips on your next steps as you carry out the plans you've made. Firstly, accept that life is unpredictable and that you will sometimes need to make adjustments to your goals. Don't beat yourself up, but rather, see this as part of the learning process. You are simply learning how to set better goals that increase your chances of success. Every time you adjust your goals, remember to evaluate them to see if they're truly SMART. Another tip is to not set yourself up for failure. People often do this by taking on too much or setting unattainable goals. To avoid this, remember to take into account your job, personal life, energy levels, and other commitments when you're deciding on how often you will work toward your goal. Try to create a feasible schedule for yourself that provides you with ample time to rest. For sustainable lifestyle changes, try to set long-term goals (as this will help you keep the big picture in mind), but break these down into smaller short-term goals (to keep yourself motivated and to more easily keep track of your progress).

Case Formulation

Another CBT technique is case formulation where you explore what factors may be causing a perceived problem to occur and what factors may be preventing these problems from being solved effectively. Case formulation considers four factors: predisposing factors, precipitating factors, perpetuating factors, and protective factors. This exercise requires you to reflect on yourself to identify possible factors in these four categories. Predisposing factors are the external or internal factors that can increase your likelihood of developing a perceived problem. These are the risk factors that apply to you (see Chapter 2). For example, your genetics, past experiences, and personality. Precipitating factors are the precise events or triggers that cause the perceived problem to present itself. For someone facing addiction, this can be anything that triggers their cravings to appear or worsen. Perpetuating factors are whatever reinforcers may be contributing and maintaining your current addiction. Protective factors are the things that can protect you against this problem, such as your personal strengths, social supports, or adaptive behavioral patterns. Reflecting on these factors can help you understand yourself more. You will see more clearly how your core beliefs, thought patterns, and present behaviors all interlink.

After this reflection, you can continue onto the next part of this exercise. For this part, you will need a paper and pen, as you will be writing down much of the reflections you've just finished. First, create a box labeled "The Problem" and within that body, write down the events and stimuli that you link to a certain problematic behavior. The second box you make should be labeled "Early Experiences." In this box, list down the experiences you had early in life that may have contributed to your problem. Draw on your previous reflections on your predisposing factors. The third box is called "Core Beliefs," and also relates to your predisposing factors, such as your personality and upbringing. In this box, write down any relevant core beliefs that you hold very strongly which may influence the problem you're facing. These beliefs may not be explicit or obvious, but you may have underlying beliefs that line several of your actions and thoughts. For example, you may believe deep down that you're a bad person or that you're never good enough.

The fourth box you will make is called "Conditional Assumptions/Rules/Attitudes" and in this box you will list the rules that you follow (either consciously or subconsciously). This box draws from your reflections on your perpetuating factors. Take some time and reflect on the things that guide your actions, that if you don't follow will make you feel uncomfortable or distressed. These rules, whether implicit or explicit, can perpetuate your negative behaviors. You may find it difficult to discover the rules that you're following, especially if they're implicit. So, here's a little tip: Rules often present themselves as if-then statements that lead you to judge yourself based on specific situations. For example, "if I don't do this perfectly, then I'm a total failure" or "if this person doesn't like me, then I must be a terrible person." Give yourself enough time to fully reflect on how you live. Dig deep and try to discover all the rules that you've set for yourself. Moving on, the fifth box is called "Maladaptive Coping Strategies," and it builds off of the previous box. Once you've written down all your rules, write down how well these rules are helping you or how badly they're hurting you. Are these rules making you a better person? Are they making you happier? Are they pushing you to be the best that you can be? Are they effective in motivating you to strive toward your goals? How do they make you feel? If you honestly answer these questions for each of your rules, you will be able to see which rules are working for you and which are working against you.

The last box is titled "Positives" and this is where you list your protective factors. In this box, write down anything that can help you deal with your problem, break the harmful cycle of thoughts and behaviors, or help you healthily cope with the thoughts and behaviors that arise in relation to your problem. Once you've filled in all these boxes, try to create a separate flowchart where you can explore how your actions and emotions are perpetuated. Think of a specific situation that produces a negative automatic thought related to your problem.

Record the emotion and actions that this thought encourages, including the bodily sensations you experience. This flowchart can help you realize your negative and unhelpful patterns. You will be able to see what drives your actions and what consequences you face due to those actions. From there, you will be able to consciously challenge those negative and maladaptive habits and replace them with things from your protective factors. All in all, this exercise helps you understand yourself and the factors impacting your current problem more. This knowledge will then make you more able to take positive actions toward your problems, by challenging your bad habits and thoughts, and replacing them with more productive coping methods.

Other Exercises

There are a few other smaller CBT exercises that can help you overcome your addiction. The first is thought records. With this exercise, you make a note of all your automatic negative thoughts and then examine them. As you're conducting this analysis, your aim is to find objective evidence that either supports or disproves those thoughts. List out all the evidence you find and compare or contrast your negative thoughts against them. This exercise can help you think more balanced, objective, fair, and kinder thoughts. By critically evaluating what you think, you avoid emotional reasoning and illogical assumptions that can increase your emotional distress and increase your cravings. One example of how thought records can help with addiction is if you have an automatic negative thought about your interaction with a friend. You may automatically assume that they're mad at you or that they don't like you. This may spark your inner insecurities, and you may consequently want to drink or indulge in your addiction to feel better. But when you record your thoughts down and critically analyze them, you may realize that you have no evidence to support your assumption and a lot of evidence that disproves it (drawing on the past experiences you've shared with this person). This may lead you to draw a more balanced and fair conclusion that you may be misinterpreting things. Or you may reason that every friendship goes through disputes and that this one instance doesn't mean that you're a bad friend or a bad person.

Behavioral experiments are another exercise you can try where you contrast negative thoughts against positive ones to observe which type of thought is more effective in changing your behavior. Often you will find that self-kindness is more effective than self-criticism. But the whole point of behavioral experiments is to figure out what form of motivation and self-direction work best for you. For example, as you're struggling to reduce your indulgence in your addiction on your recovery journey, try different approaches and observe the outcomes. You may find that you indulge less in your addiction the next time when you are hard on yourself after the last time you indulged. Or you may find that you indulge less the next time when you talk kindly to yourself after the last time. Your healing process is unique to you, so take your time to figure out what works best for you.

Finally, there is the pleasant activity schedule. This exercise entails making a weekly list of fun, enjoyable, and healthy activities that break up your daily routine. These activities should be easy, simple, and encourage positive emotions. This will help reduce your automatic negative thoughts, diminish your cravings, and keep your life interesting by breaking you away from the monotony of daily life. An example of the pleasant activity schedule at work is when you've had a long day at your job and you come back home to relax. Rather than indulging in your addiction, you can help overcome your cravings by having other fun activities planned. This activity can distract you from your cravings, fill up your time, and give you a mood boost.

These are all the CBT exercises that you can use to redirect your thoughts and subsequent actions. In the next chapter, you will learn about acceptance and commitment therapy (ACT). You will also receive several ACT exercises that can help you overcome your addiction.

CHAPTER 4

Acceptance and Commitment Therapy

Another form of therapy that is often applied on cases of addiction is acceptance and commitment therapy (ACT). This is a form of psychotherapy that emphasizes acceptance as a way to deal with negative thoughts, emotions, symptoms, or situations. In simple terms, ACT wants to help you accept what is out of your control and focus your energies instead on actions that can enrich your life. It is an empirically based psychological treatment that uses commitment, behavior change, acceptance, and mindfulness strategies to decrease the emotional distress you may feel. This can be a powerful treatment for addiction, especially if used in tandem with CBT. While CBT tackles your thoughts and negative habits, ACT can sustain, strengthen, and encourage these changes by altering your thoughts and reactions. Another way that ACT is a good treatment for addiction is found in its commitment component. Other than leading you to be more accepting toward yourself (the good and the bad), ACT encourages you to be committed to your healing process. You will become more dedicated to healthy, constructive activities that harmonize with your values and goals. This commitment will further your positive progress as you will keep working and trying to get better. You will even be able to deal with relapses better as you won't be discouraged or give up easily. Instead, you will remember your commitment, pick yourself back up, and continue facing your hardships.

The main theory behind ACT is that by increasing your acceptance of yourself, you will also increase your psychological flexibility, which will bring about a host of benefits. One of which is decreased avoidance. When you are more accepting of yourself and more mentally flexible, you will be able to confront all your thoughts, emotions, and experiences honestly, rather than habitually avoiding them. When you avoid your problems, they may simply manifest themselves in other forms in various areas of your life. So, acceptance is important to decrease your levels of avoidance, improve your psychological flexibility, and increase your courage to face uncomfortable things. Another theory behind ACT is that suffering is a natural and inescapable condition for people. Despite that, humans all have an instinctive desire to control their experiences in order to reduce the amount of suffering they have to face. Sometimes this works in your favor to reduce needless suffering. Other times, your desire for control may get out of hand and become detrimental to you, as you try to exert too much control over things or try to control things that you can't possibly control. ACT functions to help you create a rich and meaningful life alongside the inevitable experiences of pain and suffering. This is why, as previously stated, ACT works well alongside CBT, as they complement each other. CBT can help you reduce the frequency or intensity of uncomfortable and unpleasant internal experiences (such as the cognitive distortions, negative thoughts, compulsions, or urges that cause you distress). ACT can help you deal with the residual or persistent internal experiences that linger, as you're conducting CBT on yourself. This is achieved by reducing your struggle to control or completely eradicate those experiences and concurrently increasing your involvement in other meaningful life activities that are consistent with your personal values and goals. So, while CBT helps you reduce the negative internal experiences that are contributing to your addiction, it may not be able to completely erase them. This is where ACT comes in, to help you cope with the inevitable and incessant negative internal experiences that you're bound to experience throughout your life (though to varying degrees). As a result, ACT and CBT work well together to treat addiction. However, ACT also works well on its own to lower your need to control everything, increase your peace, and solidify your commitment to getting better.

There are six components to ACT that help it achieve its goals. These are:

- Acceptance: The largest and most obvious component of ACT. This means allowing your inner emotions and thoughts to occur freely. You don't try to change them, judge them, avoid them, or ignore them. This is an active process that you must consciously work at. You will be building an alternative to your instinctive avoidance or negative thoughts. You must consciously choose to allow unpleasant experiences to exist, without denying or trying to change them. This will lead to positive results in your mental health.

- Cognitive defusion: This is the process where you separate yourself from your inner experiences, allowing yourself to see your thoughts just as thoughts and nothing else. This can change how you react to your emotions and thoughts, lower the importance that your mind adds to your thoughts, and help you accept your thoughts as they are. ACT doesn't aim to limit your exposure to negative situations, but it does help you come out the other side with less fixation and fewer negative reactions to those experiences.

- Self as context: This is the process where you separate your thoughts about yourself from your actions. Often you may have judgments or perceptions about yourself that you hold to be true, without considering the evidence of your actions. You will also realize that you're not only the sum of your experiences, thoughts, or emotions. You have a self outside of whatever you're currently experiencing, so whatever happens to you cannot wholly define you. This may help you be more accepting of your life experiences.

- Being present: This involves being mindful of your surroundings and learning to live in the current moment, rather than being too focused on the past or future. You will also learn how to shift your attention toward your present experiences and away from your inner thoughts and feelings that may sometimes trap you in unproductive spirals.

- Values: ACT emphasizes the importance of knowing your values, as these are the things in your life that are important enough to you to inspire and motivate action.

This will come in handy for the commitment part of this therapy.

- Commitment: ACT will teach you various principles about how you should behave and how your current habits are harming you. Then, this form of therapy will emphasize the need for commitment to changing your negative behaviors. You will also be led to commit to actions and habits that work toward your long-term goals and correspond with your values.

ACT can help guide you through all of these components, and you will learn how to apply them in your life. You may learn how to practice acceptance, mindfulness, and cognitive defusion, or you may develop a different self-perception that goes against your negative and self-critical thoughts and feelings. You may even become more aware of when your actions don't fit your values and thus cause you mental or emotional distress. Overall, ACT can help you become more accepting, less judgmental, and more aware of your thoughts, emotions, sensations, and memories. Some of these feelings or thoughts may be new to you, as you never paid attention to them before, while some may be things that you're actively avoiding. Either way, you will learn to be more at peace with yourself and this will improve your mental health.

To talk specifically about the benefits of ACT, let's dive deeper into how your increased psychological flexibility can support your mental health. It was previously stated that ACT can improve your psychological flexibility. This is actually a great advantage to you, as psychological flexibility is your ability to embrace your thoughts and emotions when they are helpful, and to calmly set them aside when they are not. Possessing this skill will allow you to thoughtfully and rationally respond to your inner experiences, avoid impulsive behaviors or habits, and focus on living a meaningful and purposeful life. You will even be more capable of accepting and functioning with your symptoms of addiction. When your urges come up, your psychological flexibility will be able to acknowledge that they're not helpful to you and this will make it slightly easier for you to set them aside and resist them. Even if and when you relapse, your psychological flexibility will help you get through it and bounce back without beating yourself up. You will be able to realize that getting overly upset and excessively self-critical about your mistakes may only exacerbate your distress and cravings. This will help you face any relapse with aplomb and self-kindness. Now that you understand ACT more, let's start learning the exercises and skills to help you overcome your addiction.

Cognitive Defusion

As you've read, cognitive defusion is an important component of ACT. In this section, you will receive five different exercises that can help you defuse your cognition. Pick one or two that apply the most to you or that you find the most interesting, and try to practice them repeatedly over the next few days, especially when you're confronted with symptoms of addiction. And don't be discouraged if it doesn't work initially. You may need more time to practice this skill or you may need to choose a different exercise to try that works better for you. Remember to be patient and kind to yourself while trying out these exercises. If the exercises you chose initially work for you, that's great. Keep using them and practicing them. You will get better and better at cognitive defusion. If the exercises don't work initially, keep it up for a while. If they still don't work, switch things up and pick a new exercise.

The first exercise is called Your Mind. The function of this exercise is to separate yourself from your thoughts so that you can approach them more logically and be less affected by them. To do this, think of your mind as a separate entity from yourself. You can simply call this entity 'Mind.' Whenever your thoughts start to run or spiral or dip into anxiety, depression, or cravings, you can say to yourself, "There goes Mind again, chattering on" or "Wow, Mind really likes telling me that I need to do this or that, it's doing it again now" or "Yikes, Mind really needs to calm down." It may seem funny to talk about your own mind and thoughts in this way, but by treating your mind as something external rather than internal, you can create a bit of space between yourself and your negative thoughts. This can help you see your thoughts more clearly, feel a bit better, be less affected by your negative thoughts, and lower the emphasis you may place on those thoughts.

The second exercise is called Car Radio. Imagine you're sitting in the passenger seat of a car and the driver has the radio turned to an awful station. This station is playing a soundtrack of all your negative thoughts, but you're not in a position to switch the radio off or change the station. And you can't tune it out and ignore the radio because it's playing clearly inside the car. So, all you can do is tolerate the radio station and accept that these thoughts are playing, even though the noise is unpleasant.

The third exercise is called Keychain in Your Pocket. Practicing this exercise can help you accept the presence of your negative thoughts while not allowing them to control your actions. To do this activity, you must carry around a bunch of keys with you or any other bundle of things that you use often. Now, take some of your more common negative thoughts and assign them to a specific key or item in your bundle. Then, whenever you use that specific key or item, remind yourself to think the corresponding thought. After a few days of this, tell yourself that you can carry the thoughts with you, but you don't always have to think them. And even when you do think the negative thoughts, you can still use the key. This will reinforce to you that negative thoughts aren't the end of the world—your life goes on, even when you think those negative thoughts. Therefore, it's possible to carry negative thoughts and beliefs with you in life and not allow them to control your actions.

The fourth exercise is a short one called Bossy Bully. This is another practice that helps you decrease the control that your negative thoughts have on you. To do this, simply treat your negative thoughts like bullies on the playground. Ask yourself who is in charge here, you or your thoughts. You can even get a little angry at your thoughts to help you assert yourself against the bully.

The fifth and final cognitive defusion exercise is called Thoughts for Sale. In this exercise, you will distinguish between a thought that you're having and a thought that you're buying as true. Isolate whatever thought is causing you distress and then label it as fairly and objectively as you can. For example, you can label one of your thoughts as a judgment, comparison, exaggeration, criticism, and so on. Then, ask yourself what that thought is saying about you and whether or not you want to buy the thought that you are (insert relevant adjectives here, such as selfish, worthless, stupid, and so on). As with any purchase, consider what buying into this thought will cost you, and if it's truly a good and worthwhile investment.

These exercises may not alter the frequency at which you experience negative thoughts, but they are highly effective in decreasing your attachments and maladaptive reactions to particular thoughts and beliefs that aren't serving you well.

Value Clarification

Another ACT component is knowing your values. This can be hard to do, as you're not often encouraged to look inside and discover your own values. Many people live their lives just swayed by the values of others; living according to the judgments and morals of others. Here, you will be led through an exercise that can help you clarify your values, which are your heart's deepest desires for how you want to interact with and relate to yourself, others, and the world. Your values are the leading principles that guide your thoughts and actions, and motivate you as you go through life. Once you know your values, you will know what you want to do and how you want to do it. For example, you will know how you want to behave (toward your friends, family, work, environment, self, and so on), what is really deeply important to you, what you want your life to stand for, and what qualities you want to cultivate in yourself. One thing to note here is that values are not the same things as goals. Values entail ongoing action. They point you in the direction you want to go. Goals are the things you want to achieve as you move in that direction. Goals can be crossed off once they're achieved, but values will keep going forever. For example, wanting to be a good and loving partner is a value, since it involves ongoing action. Wanting to be married is a goal, as it can be achieved and crossed off, at which point it won't require any further action.

Now that you understand what values are, let's explore the exercise called the Bull's Eye. This exercise requires paper and a pen. On the paper, draw a dartboard with a bull's eye and then draw a 't' on that dartboard to divide it into four equal sections. Name those sections work/education, relationships, leisure, and personal growth/health. Now, leave that aside for now. On another piece of paper, write down your values in these four areas of life. Remember that there are no right or wrong values; everyone has different values that guide their lives. And as you're writing down your values, be careful that you don't start writing down your goals instead. To avoid this, try to think in terms of general life directions rather than specific aims and goals. On another note, you may have values that overlap and apply to two or more areas of your life. This is fine, just jot down whatever values come to you. For example, if you value psychological knowledge, this may be listed under both education and personal growth. To help yourself reflect and discover your values, you can try to ask yourself what's important to you, what you care about, what you would like to strive toward, how you would like to live your life over time, and what you would value if there were no obstacles in your way to stop you. One final thing to note as you're writing down your values is to make sure that you're writing down your own values and not the values of others. It's easy to confuse the two, as you may be used to living according to others (such as your parents, friends, siblings, mentors, teachers, and so on). So, try to take this time to really find out what personal values you have and what really matters to you.

To help you explore and clarify your personal values, here are some explanations, notes, and questions relating to each of the four areas of life:

- Work/Education: This area refers to your career, workplace (including volunteer work or other forms of unpaid work), education, knowledge, and skills development. How do you want to act toward your clients, customers, coworkers, employees, and bosses?

What personal traits and qualities do you want to bring with you to your work? What skills do you want to develop or what experiences do you want to gain from this?

- Relationships: This area of life refers to your friendships, intimacy, closeness, and special bonds in your life. This includes relationships with your friends, partner, children, parents, relatives, coworkers, and other social contacts. What type of relationships do you want to forge? How do you want to act in those relationships? What do you want to give and receive in those relationships? What personal traits and qualities do you want to develop?

- Personal Growth/Health: This area of life refers to your continual development as a person. This entails your creativity, religion, spirituality, life skills, meditation, connection to nature, exercise, nutrition, mental health, social health, and so on. This also includes dealing with your health risk factors, such as smoking or addiction. Which areas of your personal growth do you want to focus on the most? Why are those areas important to you?

- Leisure: This area of life refers to how you relax, enjoy, play, or stimulate yourself. This has to do with your hobbies or whatever activities you do for rest, creativity, fun, and recreation. Which leisure activities would you like to increase in your life? Which leisure activities make you feel the happiest and healthiest?

Once you've written down your values for these four areas of life, return to your bull's eye and make an X in each of the four quadrants. The X represents where you stand currently, along with how well you're living in harmony with your own values in those areas of life. The closer your X is to the middle of the board (the bull's eye), the better you're living fully by your values in that area of life. Marking these Xs can help you see which areas of your life are going well according to your values, and which areas of your life are a bit far off the mark. This can then lead you to know which areas of your life deserve more attention. And since you've clarified your values already, you will have a clearer picture of what actions and changes need to be done.

Mindfulness

The last ACT skill you will learn here is mindfulness, which is the practice of being more fully aware of your present moment rather than judging it, dwelling on the past, or worrying about the future. Mindfulness exercises typically involve bringing your attention to your sensory stimuli to ground yourself more in the present moment. For example, if you're experiencing negative thoughts or urges that are causing you discomfort and unease, you are encouraged to use mindfulness to bring yourself back to the present, focus on your surroundings rather than your thoughts and emotions, and significantly reduce your distress.

Other than the exercises you will be led through, there are daily habits and practices you can use to cultivate mindfulness in your everyday routine. Here are the suggestions for how you can focus on the present moment, quiet your inner chaos, and attain mindfulness:

- Pay attention: Slow down and take some time to notice things around you, such as your own feelings, thoughts (without judging them or obsessing over them), senses (focus on all five senses), and the things in the world around you. Try to enjoy the things you're currently experiencing (such as a cool breeze or a good meal).

- Focus on the moment: Don't waste time regretting the past, which you can't change, or worrying about the future, which you can't control or predict. Rather, just experience whatever is happening to you right now. This can reduce your emotional distress and keep you grounded in what's real and within your control.

- Try mindfulness meditation: You will receive some guidance on how to do mindfulness meditation later. If you regularly practice this exercise, you will receive countless benefits on your mental and physical health. Even if you have trouble staying still and focused initially during meditation, take comfort in the fact that you're not alone. Mindfulness isn't something that's easily attainable. You have to practice and keep working at it.

- Try mindfulness activities: If meditation doesn't work too well for you, there are many other activities that can ease you into the practice of mindfulness. For example, gardening, cleaning the house, grocery shopping, or listening to music can all be activities that train your mindfulness if you adopt the right approach. As you're doing these activities and any others that you think are appropriate for mindfulness, try to focus on the present and quiet your thoughts. Rather than paying attention to your thoughts that normally run wild—giving incessant commentary on what you're doing, what you've done, what you should be doing, and so on—gently bring your attention back to the present. The goal here isn't to silence or suppress your thoughts, but simply to quiet them, observe them without judgment, and to gently refocus on your present activity.

- Try an app: With all the technology available to you now, it would be a shame not to use it. So, try using an app for mindfulness. There are many good options out there that offer you information, resources, and guidance for becoming more mindful.

- Focus on one thing at a time: Multitasking is a counterproductive habit, as you may become distracted and not work efficiently on either task. Instead, try to just concentrate on a single task completely.

- Go for a walk: Spending time outdoors is a great way to ground yourself in the current moment, as you will be surrounded by new stimuli that you can concentrate on. There will be new sights, sounds, smells, and sensations in the world around you, so focus on your senses.

- Be kind to yourself: The whole point of mindfulness is to be nonjudgmental, so remind yourself not to be harsh or critical when you find your mind wandering during mindfulness exercises. You must accept yourself and your flaws, treating yourself with kindness and compassion.

Aside from these general daily practices, mindfulness can also be cultivated through meditation exercises which can be practiced about once a week or more, according to your energy and time constraints. The one mindfulness meditation exercise you will learn here is called Body Scan Meditation. This exercise can release your physical tension and ground yourself in the present moment. In this exercise, you will gradually bring your attention to each part of your body and notice all your bodily sensations, including your tension, discomfort, aches, pains, numbness, and so on. The goal of this exercise isn't to relieve your pain entirely, but to become aware of it so that you can better manage it. It's recommended that you practice this meditation every day in order to reap more benefits, but it can be time consuming and tiring, so try to do it only as much as you're able to. It doesn't need to be every day, but try to aim for at least once a week. The primary benefits of this meditation are stress reduction, reduced fatigue, reduced inflammation, and reduced insomnia. These emotional and physical benefits can help break or alleviate the cycle of physical and psychological tension that tends to perpetuate itself. This meditation can also help you achieve and maintain a more relaxed state.

The steps to follow for Body Scan Meditation are as follows:

1. Sit or lie down in a comfortable position. Take a few deep breaths and let your breathing rest at a natural pace.

2. Start breathing from your belly rather than from your

chest, allowing your abdomen to expand and contract as you take each breath.

3. Bring your awareness to your feet and start to observe the sensations you have in your feet. Notice and acknowledge any pains and accompanying emotions and thoughts. Don't judge any of this, but simply breathe through it. Breathe into the tension, focus on your sensations, and continue breathing. Observe what happens. Visualize the tension leaving your body as you exhale on each breath. Imagine the tension being expelled and evaporating into the air. Give yourself enough time to observe your sensations in this body part. When you're ready, move onto the next body part, slowly working your way up.

4. In this way, scan your entire body, moving up from your feet to the top of your head. Notice how you're feeling and where you feel the most stress. Breathe through whatever tightness, pain, pressure, or discomfort you may feel. This will help you release the tension in your body. In the future, you will also be more aware of these sensations, so you will be alerted to them and able to release them.

The more you practice this exercise, the easier it will become. This meditation can increase your body awareness, stress management, and relaxation, so you should try to practice it often. It's a great way to address both your physical and mental distress. In the next chapter, you will learn about yet another type of therapy used to treat addiction: exposure and response prevention therapy.

CHAPTER 5

Exposure and Response Prevention Therapy

Another form of therapy that can address your symptoms of addiction is exposure and response prevention (ERP) therapy. This treatment method is especially useful in helping you cope with the triggers that spark your cravings for your addiction. Essentially, you will be led to face those triggers and subsequent obsessive thoughts, emotional distress, negative experiences, and compulsions that often push you to indulge in your addiction. Through ERP, you will learn to face those triggers without consequently indulging in your addiction. You will start slow, with situations or triggers that cause you tolerable distress or anxiety. Gradually, you will build up a higher tolerance to deal with your triggers. This end goal is achieved by the two components of ERP, that is exposure and response prevention. The exposure component entails exposing yourself to the thoughts, objects, situations, and images that make you anxious or trigger your addiction. The response prevention component entails making a conscious choice not to engage with your addiction once your negative thoughts and emotions have been triggered. If you struggle with addiction, you may have tried exposing yourself to your triggers in an effort to resist them. If you've done this before, then chances are that you only saw your anxiety spike and ended up engaging in your addiction. With ERP, you will essentially be doing the same thing, but with two key differences that will increase your chances of success. Namely, you will start with low-level triggers that are more manageable, and you will have made a decisive commitment prior to the exposure that you will not give in and engage with your addiction. This will help you reduce the amount of time you allow your triggers to provoke your addiction, and over time, those triggers will start affecting you less and less.

Another way to understand ERP is to think of your responses to your triggers as an alarm system. Your triggers may cause you to lean into your addiction as a way to cope with certain emotions, thoughts, or situations. When faced with those undesirable or uncomfortable things, your alarm goes off to get your attention and spur you to do something to protect yourself. But the thing about alarm systems is that they can't distinguish between real or perceived threats. Whether it's a robber breaking into your house or a bird landing on the roof, your alarm system will sound. What you will be teaching yourself through ERP is to distinguish between real or perceived threats. Just because your alarm sounds, doesn't mean that you must act as if you're really being threatened. Often, you assume your body is right, experience the consequent negative thoughts and emotions, and then indulge in your addiction. ERP aims to break this cycle by having you stop and consider whether you're really in danger or not. When you indulge in your addiction every time you're faced with your triggers, you reinforce to your brain that those triggers can only be dealt with through your addiction. This will only fuel your reliance on your addiction. So, to reduce your reliance and vulnerability to your triggers, you must make the decision to stop being controlled by your compulsions and urges. This will gradually change how your brain responds to your triggers and your alarm system, anxiety, and emotional distress will become more in line with what you're actually experiencing.

It's been briefly stated how ERP has two components. Now, let's delve deeper into how these components can help you with your addiction. The exposure component of ERP makes use of a behavioral principle called habituation. This is the process by which your behavioral and sensory responses diminish over time, through repeated exposure to a specific stimulus.

Everyone has experienced habituation before. If you've ever noticed a new smell in a room and eventually stopped noticing it, that's habituation. Your olfactory sensors note the new stimulus, but after being exposed to it for a longer period of time, they will stop noting it and put it in the background. Or if you've ever jumped into a pool with cold water, but after a few minutes you don't notice the cold anymore, that's also habituation. Another example is if you live near an airport, train station, or busy highway. Initially, you may have had trouble sleeping through all the noise, but after some time you will have gotten used to it as your sensory neurons simply stopped noting and reacting to the noise. So, your senses can become habituated to various types of stimuli. Exposure therapy takes advantage of this principle by repeatedly exposing you to your triggers so that habituation can occur. This can be seen as intentional habituation. Over time, the intensity of the exposure is slowly increased. As this occurs, you will continually allow yourself to experience the emotional distress until it subsides (and it will subside as you become habituated).

The exposure component of ERP can be conducted through real life exposure to your triggers or by imagined exposure (where you create thought experiments in your mind). Either way, you will repeatedly face your trigger situations until habituation occurs and your compulsive responses are diminished and eventually extinguished. This concept of an ever decreasing response to your triggers is based on the principle of classical conditioning or learning theory. This principle demonstrates how you can learn to be less affected or afraid of neutral stimuli (that is, stimuli that don't pose an actual, real threat to your safety). Your fear, anxiety, and emotional distress will spike when paired association forms between a fear-inducing stimuli and a neutral, conditioned stimulus. These reactions will be diminished and eliminated by reversing that process and association. In other words, you will reduce and unlearn your reactions to your triggers by uncoupling the paired association between your fear (and emotional distress) and the neutral, conditioned stimulus. Whatever your triggers are that cause you distress and increase your urges for your addiction, you will face those situations until habituation occurs. This suggests that your triggers, which were fear-inducing stimuli, will no longer produce fearful or distressing reactions, meaning that the association between your trigger and your distress has been undone. Therefore, your negative reactions and subsequent reliance on your addiction will be diminished. After some time and repeated exposure, you will learn something new: That nothing bad usually comes from your triggers.

The next component of ERP is response prevention. If you're struggling with addiction, then you may have developed ritualized and repetitive behaviors in response to your triggers. These behaviors are known as your compulsions and urges to engage in your addiction. These behaviors serve to neutralize the negative reactions you experience when faced with your triggers. Since these behaviors reduce your experience of those negative reactions and since your addiction invariably brings you short-term pleasure, your compulsions may feel intrinsically rewarding. Therefore, they are often repeated, reinforced, and indulged in. Response prevention aims to combat this cycle and is also based on a principle of learning theory, that is the principle of operant conditioning. This principle states that when a behavior is no longer reinforced or rewarded, it fades away and becomes extinct. So, the less you indulge in your addiction as a response to your triggers, the weaker and less frequent your compulsions will become. Indulging in your addiction may also be construed as escape or avoidance behaviors and they have the same rewarding function as compulsive rituals. They are protective coping strategies that address your anxiety and emotional distress in the short-term. You may momentarily decrease your emotional distress by escapism or avoidance, and since it feels good to alleviate your stress quickly, those behaviors are rewarded and reinforced. Whether you're indulging in your addiction as a form of compulsive behavior, escapism, or avoidance behavior, you will feel rewarded in the short-term and thus reinforce your addiction in the long-term. You can only eliminate these reinforced behaviors (that is, your indulgence in your addiction) by preventing these behaviors. By preventing these behaviors, you prevent them from being rewarded, thus preventing them from being reinforced. Once a behavior is no longer rewarded, it is no longer reinforced, and it will eventually stop. Therefore, response prevention is a vital component of ERP, along with the exposure component. Together, they form an effective treatment response for addiction.

Before you embark on conducting ERP, you must ensure that you're willing to tolerate some discomfort during the habituation process. This willingness will make you more prepared in advance of the therapy. You shouldn't feel forced or coerced into any situation with ERP, as this may only aggravate your addiction by exposing you to more than you're ready to handle. And even if you're not coerced into anything, it's okay to stop the process whenever it feels impossible or too difficult to complete an exercise. When this happens, extend yourself some grace, understanding, kindness, and patience. Calmly try to assess what happened, adjust the exercise accordingly, ready your mind, and try again.

Other things to clear up before starting ERP are the common misconceptions about it. Firstly, let's define how ERP is different from traditional psychotherapy (or talk therapy).

Psychotherapy typically aims to improve your addiction by helping you gain insight into your problems. This can be very helpful for certain psychological conditions and for dealing with the emotions and thoughts that cause or are caused by your addiction. However, aside from the mental and psychological parts of your addiction, there is also a very real active and physical part where your compulsions and urges can sometimes control you. This is where ERP comes in. It may not address your psychological issues as extensively as psychotherapy, but ERP can help you address the physical symptoms of your addiction. Moving on, a common myth about ERP is that it's simply the same as facing your fears. This isn't true as, though facing your fears can be part of ERP, this form of therapy involves a lot more than just that. With ERP, you are not only facing your fears, but also practicing resistance to your habitual responses (that is, indulgence in your addiction). If ERP were simple facing your fears, your cycles of addiction may only be perpetuated. It's because you're facing your fears while practicing response prevention that you're able to learn new ways of dealing with your triggers.

Another myth is that ERP is the same as flooding. Flooding is another treatment method that aims to reset your nervous system by immersing you in your feared situations. This may often overwhelm your senses. With flooding, you're meant to stay in those overwhelming situations until your anxiety and fear reduce to normal levels. This is a rather extreme treatment method that should only be applied in specific situations and with the guidance of a mental health professional. These professionals are the best equipped to determine whether flooding would be helpful or harmful to you. If it works, it can help you achieve great progress, though it will be incredibly challenging and demanding on your mind and body. If it doesn't work, you may be unnecessarily exposing yourself to intense emotional discomfort and distress, and you may spark a spiral into your addiction. In conclusion, flooding shouldn't be administered by yourself. Now that you understand what flooding is, you should be able to see how it differs from ERP. With flooding, you're thrown into the deep end of the pool. With ERP, you start in the kiddy pool and slowly work your way toward the deep end.

Creating a Trigger Ladder

Now that you have sufficient information about ERP to safely conduct it on yourself, let's get into the nitty gritty details of how to effectively do it. The first step is to make a list of your triggers or anything else (situations, objects, thoughts, images, places) that provoke your addiction. For example, if stress is a common trigger for your addiction, you may include: having many work projects that are undone, having many work emails you need to reply to, having a lot of chores you need to get done, and so on. Or if social situations are a common trigger, you may include: greeting a coworker, asking a stranger a question, eating lunch with a friend, or calling someone on the phone. A useful thing to do once you've written down all your triggers is to group them together. Try to find a common theme that links a few of your triggers into one group. You should have a few different groups of fears from your list of triggers. For example, you may find that a lot of triggers have to do with loneliness, stress, boredom, relationships, and so on. So, to help you get more organized, group your triggers into different themes so that you have a list of triggers for each theme.

Step two is to build a trigger ladder for each theme. With all the triggers you have listed under each theme, arrange them from the least triggering to the most triggering. To do this, try to rate every item on your list on a scale of zero to ten, depicting how strongly they affect you and cause you to indulge in your addiction. Once you're rated each situation, you can use those ratings to help you arrange your triggers in ascending order. When building a trigger ladder, it's important to identify a specific goal for that theme of triggers (for example, for the theme of social anxiety triggers, you can have the goal of eating a meal at a restaurant). This specific goal will help you determine the steps you need to achieve that goal, starting from the least triggering and slowly progressing you to reach your goal. For example, you can start by getting a coffee at a coffee shop, then having a snack at a sparsely populated diner, then having a snack at the restaurant and sitting near the door, then having a meal at the restaurant and sitting in the middle of the room. Of course, this may be harder to do for certain themes, so though having a specific goal is recommended, you can also have a general goal. For example, for the theme of stress triggers, you can simply have the goal of not indulging in your addiction whenever you have a stressful day or a stressful thought. Then, you can simply arrange your list of stress triggers in ascending order (they don't have to all be around the same action like the restaurant example). This will still help you deal with your stress triggers more productively. Remember that you will have many themes of triggers, so be sure to build separate ladders for each theme. Some of these themes will have specific goals, while others can have more general goals. Either way, the constant trait is that you will start with the triggers that cause you the least urges and compulsions, and then slowly work your way up to the most triggering situations. It's important to be patient and not skip steps on your ladder. Start small and take gradual steps.

To help you take smaller steps, some of your trigger situations can be broken down into smaller ones. For example, if talking to your coworkers triggers your addiction, you can face this challenge by breaking it up into smaller steps. Start by greeting them in the morning, then asking them a quick question next time, and eventually try to strike up a full conversation with them. As you're building your trigger ladder, you can make certain situations more or less challenging by considering a few factors. Firstly, consider the length of time you want to expose yourself to your trigger. Second, consider the time of day you want to confront your trigger, as this may make it more approachable or scary. Third, consider the environment, as this may affect how strongly you're triggered. Fourth, consider the company you're in, as this may make any situation more or less triggering. These are a few examples of the factors to consider when making your trigger ladder. With these considerations in mind, you can tweak your trigger situations to make them easier or harder for yourself.

Step three in creating an exposure ladder is to face your fears, that is to expose yourself to the items on your trigger list. Start with the trigger that causes you the least emotional distress and repeatedly engage in that situation until you start to feel less anxious about it. Be repetitive and consistent about this by staying in the situation for a prolonged amount of time or repeating the action several times. If you stay in a situation for long enough or repeatedly engage in an activity enough times, your anxiety and emotional distress will start to reduce. The longer you face something, the more habituated you will become and the less energy you will have to react negatively toward it. Eventually, your negative feelings will fade and you will react less extremely the next time you encounter the situation. A useful tip to follow as you're doing this third step is to track your levels of emotional distress (such as your compulsions, urges, or anxiety) during your exposure and to keep trying to remain in those situations until your levels of distress decrease by about half. For example, if you rated calling a friend as a six out of ten on your trigger scale, try to stay on the call during your exposure until you can confidently and fairly assess your current distress levels as a three out of ten.

Other tips on conducting your exposures are to plan your exposure exercises in advance and to track your progress. Planning these exercises in advance can help you feel more in control and lower your stress levels. So, try to plan in advance what you will do and when. As for tracking your progress, try to identify how you felt before and after your exposure exercise. This can help you see more clearly how your emotions are progressing. You can even write down things you learned from each exposure experience. Finally, an important thing to remember as you're doing your exposure exercises is to not rush. Facing your fears is a scary and harrowing task, so be patient with yourself and take your time. Being impatient and rushing through your trigger ladder may cause you to relapse into your addiction and cause you much more harm than good. So, go at a pace that you can manage, and you will surely see slow and steady improvements.

The fourth step for ERP is to practice on a regular basis. As you're facing each step on your ladder, be sure to repeat your exposure exercises daily or at least weekly. The more often you practice, the faster your fear will fade. More practice will also help you maintain the progress you've made. Even if you've gotten used to something, your old fears and negative reactions may come back, so remember to keep exposing yourself to it every now and then. An important aspect of practicing ERP is to re-rate your entire trigger ladder every once in a while. As you're exposing yourself to your triggers, your trigger ratings may shift and change. So, to keep your trigger ladder updated and relevant, remember to re-rate it. This can help you see the progress you've made and help you identify which steps of your ladder need more attention and which can be removed. Keep in mind that all exposures should be planned, prolonged, and repeated.

Finally, the fifth step of ERP is to reward brave behavior. It's not easy to face your fears or to resist the temptations of your addiction. So, be sure to reward yourself when you do it. Give yourself specific rewards to motivate yourself. For example, promise to buy yourself a treat, such as booking or engaging in an enjoyable activity once you reach your goals. Another form of reward is positive self-talk. Remember to give rewards that correspond to your level of achievement. Give yourself smaller rewards for achieving the lower-rated goals and bigger rewards for the higher-rated goals. And don't be discouraged if you're stuck on a single step for a while or if your fears creep back. This can happen sometimes and it's very normal. Just keep practicing, plan your exposures, and maybe break that step into smaller steps.

This is how you can conduct ERP on yourself. Remember to be patient and kind to yourself as you do this. In the next chapter, you will learn about relapses and how to handle them.

CHAPTER 6

Relapses in Your Healing Process

Relapses are to be expected, as you're recovering from an addiction. However, this expectation is only meant to decrease the emotional distress you may feel in response to a relapse. It is not meant to decrease your vigilance or wariness of relapses. Of course, you should do your best to prevent any relapses. You would never want to regress on all the progress you've made. But you should also be ready to deal with relapses when they occur. That is, through the skills you've trained with CBT and ACT, you must try to be kind, accepting, and understanding with yourself if you ever do relapse. What's important is not the past mistakes you've made, but your current decisions on how to move forward. So, if you ever relapse, don't focus on beating yourself up over it. Rather, focus your energies on bouncing back and continuing on your healing journey. The skills you need to do this are covered in the previous chapters on therapy treatments. And now, in this chapter, you will focus your attention instead on relapse prevention.

To better prepare yourself to prevent a relapse, you must first understand what a relapse is. Relapse is more of a process than an event. There are a few stages you go through before you eventually revert to your habits of addiction. The first stage is the emotional relapse, followed by a mental relapse, and finally ending with a physical relapse. For the first stage of emotional relapse, this may occur when you remember your last relapse or when you think about how you don't want to relapse or fall into addiction again. At this stage, you're not thinking about indulging in your addiction again, but your emotions and consequent behaviors are starting to lay the foundation for a relapse. At this stage, you may not be planning to relapse, so you may not notice that you're at risk of a relapse. This ignorance or denial can prevent you from taking the necessary measures to prevent the progression of a relapse. Some signs that you're experiencing emotional relapse are isolation, talking less to your friends and family, not attending or speaking in meetings, focusing on the problems of others, trouble sleeping, and poor eating habits. If you think you're in an emotional relapse, you should focus on two main goals. First, re-emphasize to yourself the importance of self-care. Second, try to recognize that your ignorance or denial is preventing you from taking positive action to prevent a relapse.

The next stage is mental relapse, where you are internally struggling between your desire to remain abstinent and your desire to indulge in your addiction again. If you're not sure whether you're in a mental relapse or not, try to notice whether or not you're craving your addiction, thinking about the things or places or people associated with your addiction in the past, exaggerating the positive parts of your past addiction, minimizing the negative parts of your past addiction, lying, bargaining, trying to plan how you can indulge in your addiction while still remaining in control, looking for chances to relapse, or planning a relapse. If you're experiencing any of these signs, you are probably at an increased risk of a physical relapse, especially during special events (such as holidays, social gatherings, or trips) where you may try to justify indulging in your addiction again. As you're recovering from an addiction, it's normal to think about indulging in your addiction again. You will occasionally think about and crave your past addiction. This is a normal part of recovery that you must be aware of in order to protect yourself and ready yourself to combat those cravings and challenges.

Finally, there is the physical relapse, where you resume using the substance of your addiction. This may be an initial use or a full blown regression into your past addiction. If you have a history of addiction, you may have difficulty controlling how much you use, so even an initial use of the substance may lead to more if you don't correct yourself. Physical relapses often occur when you believe your relapse won't be noticed.

Potential Causes of Relapses

Now that you know the stages of a relapse, let's explore the causes. There are 10 common triggers for addiction relapses. The most obvious is withdrawal. Many people relapse within their first week of stopping due to the withdrawal symptoms they experience. Even if you get past the first week, there are still acute withdrawal symptoms that can last for up to 6 to 18 months. Depending on the type of substance used, the amount you used, the frequency at which you used it, and how long your addiction has been going on for, your withdrawal symptoms will vary in intensity. Some common withdrawal symptoms are nausea, cold sweats, vomiting, diarrhea, restlessness, insomnia, and muscle aches. So, if you're recovering from substances that have intense withdrawal symptoms, it's highly recommended that you seek a medical detox where you can safely rid your body of the substance.

The second cause of relapses is your mental health. Often, your addiction may have developed as a way to cope with your mental health concerns. Once you remove your addiction, you will need to cope with those concerns on your own. This will require long-term attention to sustain your recovery. If you only focus on physical healing and don't address your mental health, you will be at an increased risk of a relapse.

The third cause of relapses is people. People with addiction often surround themselves with likeminded people who support and encourage their addiction. This can be dangerous when you're recovering. Seeing them engaging in your past addiction or hearing them encourage you to re-engage with your addiction may trigger a relapse. On that note, part of your healing process should be to surround yourself with people who truly want the best for you, and to set healthy boundaries with your friends and family. Don't intentionally surround yourself with people who are indulging in your past addiction unless you're confident that you have a stable foundation in your own recovery.

Fourthly, places may also trigger your addiction. Any place that you associate with your addiction should be avoided, at least initially. For example, these places may come in the form of bars, casinos, parties, and so on. The place will be dependent on each individual and their specific addiction. You must be extra aware of this potential trigger, as you may unconsciously associate certain places with your addiction, and so you may find yourself being adversely affected without knowing why. It's important to keep reflecting and asking yourself what potential triggers you may have. In the same vein, things may trigger your addiction. This can be anything you associate with your addiction, such as glasses clinking, the feel of money, credit cards, or pill bottles. Whatever you associate with your addiction is something to be mindful of. Though it's virtually impossible to avoid all these things, simply being aware of them can help you be more mindful and understanding of why you may be affected by certain things. This will then give you the opportunity to choose how you want to respond and cope.

Poor self-care is another potential cause for a relapse. When you're enacting proper self-care, you will feel better about yourself and have better mental health. On the flip side, poor self-care will decrease your mental health and happiness, and potentially trigger a relapse. For example, poor nutrition and sleep-hygiene can cause physical, emotional, and mental damage that will lower your mood, increase your distress, and increase your cravings for your addiction. Moving on, relationships and intimacy can spur a relapse. If you weren't in a relationship when you entered recovery, it's recommended that you abstain from one for several months until you're more stable in your recovery. This is to prevent you from using your partner to fill the void left by your addiction. Another reason to avoid relationships in the initial stages of your recovery is that, if your addiction was to alcohol, dating and intimacy will most probably expose you to alcohol, and you may not know how to handle those situations. Both new and long-term relationships (that existed even prior to recovery) can trigger unpleasant and undesirable emotions that may increase your distress and cravings for your addiction. All in all, relationships can expose you to a variety of experiences that you're not ready to cope with or navigate through just yet.

The eighth cause of relapses is pride or overconfidence. You may erroneously believe that you will never indulge in your addiction again no matter what. You may not be having any cravings right now and simply be enjoying your recovery. You may have a clear memory of the negative effects you suffered from your addiction. All this can make you very confident in your recovery, but it's important to remember that everyone is vulnerable to relapses. So, don't be so confident that you put yourself in risky situations. Don't try to prove anything to yourself or others, and don't be complacent or prideful. No matter how confident you feel, you must realistically assess what's best for you now and avoid any needless temptations. The ninth cause of relapses is boredom or isolation. Your addiction probably took up a lot of your time, so now that you're sober, you may realize that you have a lot of free time. This can make you feel bored, isolated, or lonely. These emotions may then cause you to have negative thoughts and emotions which trigger your cravings for your addiction. While it's not healthy to overbook yourself in an attempt to escape reality and avoid your thoughts, it's also not healthy to be alone and isolated during early recovery. So, try to engage in some healthy behaviors (such as exercise or your hobbies) and spend more time with your loved ones.

The tenth and final cause of relapses are uncomfortable emotions. You probably engaged in your addiction when you felt tired, angry, sad, lonely, stressed, and so on. Now that you're without your addiction, you must find ways to cope with these emotions on your own. Learn to be more aware of these emotions, accept them, and cope with them. This can be achieved through the skills taught to you in CBT and ACT.

Relapse Prevention

So far, you've learned the stages of relapse and the potential causes. This information will help you understand relapses better and make you more aware and vigilant. With that being said, the final piece of the puzzle for you to receive is information on relapse prevention. This way, you can both notice your risk of a relapse and take action to prevent it. There are four main strategies that you can use to support yourself in relapse prevention. These are therapy, medications, monitoring, and peer support. Try to take advantage of as many of these as you can to decrease your chances of a relapse.

The first strategy you can use is therapy. Several forms of therapy are used to help people overcome addiction. You've explored three of these within this book alone. There are many other forms that you can use and combine to treat your addiction. Some of these therapies can be administered on your own (as long as you have sufficient knowledge and proper guidance), while others must be done with a mental health professional. Motivational interviewing is one such therapy that must be done with a therapist. This approach aims to increase your readiness and willingness to change destructive behavior. To do this, the therapist employs several techniques such as discussing your concerns, focusing and guiding the discussion, evoking motivation and confidence in your ability to change, and helping you plan to change by developing a series of steps that you can use. This requires an outsider's objective and informed point of view to help you explore your inner thoughts and emotions, and so a mental health professional is required for this form of therapy. There's also contingency management which requires not only a mental health professional, but a recovery center too. This form of therapy applies operant conditioning to your recovery. For example, when you check yourself into a center and submit a negative urine drug screen, you may receive motivational incentives such as certain foods or privileges. This form of therapy is highly effective in the short-term, though for long-term recovery, you will need to rely on other forms of therapy.

Two forms of therapy that you can do with a therapist or on your own are CBT and ACT. CBT is widely used to treat addiction, as it can help you overcome the challenges that perpetuate your addiction and equip you with the skills you need to sustain your recovery. ACT is also used to treat addiction, as it can help you change your relationship with the substance of your addiction. There's also the community reinforcement approach that emphasizes the benefits of sobriety and reduces the positive reinforcement of your addiction. This form of therapy promotes family involvement to achieve this.

Other than therapy, you can make use of medications in your recovery process. The relevant medications are different depending on the substance of your addiction. For nicotine, the relevant medications usually target cessation rather than relapse prevention, but they are still effective in helping you with your recovery. One medication that's effective for relapse prevention with nicotine is bupropion. For alcohol addiction, naltrexone can be used to help reduce your cravings and thus prevent relapses. Acamprosate is another medication that can help prevent you from using alcohol and relapsing. For opioid addiction, buprenorphine is a partial opioid agonist that can reduce your risk of a relapse. For methamphetamine addiction, antidepressants, antipsychotics, oxytocin, gabapentin, and other medications have been shown to help prevent relapses. Overall, there is a variety of medication available to you to help you prevent relapses. These medications should only be taken once advised to by a medical professional. Don't medicate yourself based on your own limited knowledge, as this may exacerbate your addiction.

Furthermore, monitoring is another strategy to prevent relapses. There are various forms of monitoring that can be used to detect substance abuse. You can schedule regular monitoring with trusted loved ones to hold yourself accountable to your abstinence. Objective evidence of abstinence is a critical part of relapse prevention. Proving your sobriety can allow you to reward yourself (thus reinforcing your positive habits and increasing your commitment to abstinence). Knowing that you will be tested can also serve as a deterrent against relapses or fantasizing about relapses. Urine drug screens are widely used as a form of monitoring and can detect a wide variety of substances. However, these screens cost money and time, as you need to travel to a clinic or testing center and pay for the testing materials and staff time. Point-of-care tests usually use drug test strips or cups that can give you your results in about five minutes. Laboratory tests take significantly longer and cost more, but they do offer higher sensitivity and specificity. For people suffering from alcohol addiction, breathalyzers are often used. This is a quick and inexpensive form of monitoring. However, it's specific to alcohol and can't detect any other substance. Then, there's also saliva tests and hair follicle drug tests that can be used to detect certain drugs, but these aren't widely used in treatment. Other than monitoring for substances, you can also ask your loved ones to monitor your behavior. If they're informed on the warning signs of relapses, they will be able to alert you when you're acting strangely and help you take action to prevent a relapse.

Moreover, peer support is an important strategy in your efforts to prevent a relapse. Many peer support programs have been developed to create a community of people who share the same experiences and can support each other. Often, those who have progressed in recovery are there to help those in the earlier stage of recovery. The most widely known peer support program is Alcoholics Anonymous (AA). This program emphasizes how attending frequent meetings with other fellow alcoholics, working through a specific program, and receiving guidance and friendship from a mentor can help you recover and sustain your progress. Sharing your experiences with other people who can relate to what you're going through can help you create a safe, supportive environment for yourself that will facilitate your healing. Seeing how so many others are suffering and struggling to overcome addiction with you can also motivate you to maintain your progress and keep you moving forward. Other than these groups, peer support can also be used in the form of peer recovery coaches. Such individuals have experienced the same addiction as you and have been abstinent for a long time (usually one or two years). Peer recovery coaches complete around 40 hours of training and a specified amount of hours in the field before they are certified as coaches. After that, they can work one-on-one with clinics or at offices with assigned individuals. Other than these formal methods of peer support, there is also the simple path of relying on your loved ones for comfort, care, advice, and help. As you're fighting your addiction, the last thing you should do is isolate yourself. Instead of pulling back from the people who want to help you, try to embrace them. Teach them how they can help you and treat you as you're going through this. They may not always get it right, but if they keep learning and you keep communicating with them, eventually you will build a strong and healthy support system.

Now that you're well equipped to fend off potential relapses, let's move onto the next chapter, where you will learn how to build healthy relationships with others.

CHAPTER 7

Building Healthy Relationships During Your Recovery Process

The relationships you have can significantly impact your recovery process. They can support and comfort you, or they can increase your emotional distress and chances of a relapse. So, when you're trying to abstain from your addiction, it's vital to develop positive and healthy relationships that will support you and reduce your emotional distress, thus preventing you from relapsing. Developing healthy relationships applies to your current social network and the new people you meet along your recovery journey.

The first, most basic step in building healthy relationships that will support your recovery is to avoid toxic relationships. When you're struggling with addiction, it may get to a point where your primary relationship is with the substance of your addiction. As your symptoms intensify, you may find yourself spending more and more time and effort in relation to your substance of choice. You may find yourself obsessing over how to indulge more in your addiction or spending all your time engaged in it. This means that you may have neglected your healthy relationships and formed more toxic ones with other addicts who support your addiction. Maintaining these relationships in the beginning stages of your recovery can be detrimental, as you may be pressured back into your addiction. Even if they don't pressure you, simply hanging out with those you associate with your addiction can push you to return to your old habits.

Other than that, there are many different ways that a relationship can be toxic. A toxic relationship can contaminate your self-esteem, happiness, worldview, and commitment to recovery. All the emotional damage that comes from that toxic relationship will push you to seek comfort and safety in your addiction. If you're stuck in a toxic relationship, you need to do what's best for yourself and leave. If it's someone you can't exactly cut off and stop seeing (such as a family member or a mutual friend), you can try to limit your time with them and emotionally distance yourself from them. There are a few ways you can tell if you're in a toxic relationship. Firstly, you will feel on edge whenever you're around them, always braced for some repercussions. Their questions, statements, looks, and gestures may all be traps or ways to tell you that you've done something wrong. And this doesn't come from a loving, forgiving place where they want the best for you. Instead, it comes from an accusatory, superior place where they just want to levy guilt and shame against you. Another sign that you're in a toxic relationship is if you avoid saying what you want or need, since you feel like there's no point. Everyone has needs in relationships, whether that's connection, love, validation, appreciation, affection, and so on. But some relationships neglect those needs, ignore them, or even mock them. If your attempts to communicate and meet your own needs in a relationship are met with hostility, violence, or accusations (of neediness, insecurity, jealousy, or insanity), then it's a toxic relationship.

Next, if the other person puts in no effort to maintain or improve the relationship, you can feel free to walk away. If all the effort, love, and compromise is coming from you, and if you're the only one investing in the relationship, then ask yourself what you're benefiting from this relationship. This may seem like a selfish question, but it's never selfish to take care of yourself. Human relationships are built on reciprocity. If you're the only one making an effort, it can be exhausting (emotionally, mentally, and physically) and lonely. And no matter what you believe, you will never do enough to make them more invested.

Their lack of effort is not a comment on you, but on them. On the other hand, they can be involved in the relationship in a toxic way. For example, if you're not allowed to say no in the relationship. Healthy relationships require respect for each other's needs and wants. They should be able to withstand a 'no' now and then. If your partner gets mad or reacts negatively or you somehow get punished whenever you say no, then they're not being respectful or reasonable.

A more subtle way that a relationship can be toxic is if they don't support you. A relationship is a joint effort where you're a team and you're working toward the same goal. However, a toxic relationship won't give you much support. You will feel like you're alone in all your battles and struggles. A more obvious way to spot a toxic relationship is abuse. This can be physical, verbal, mental, emotional, or psychological. Any form of abuse is unacceptable, and you must find the courage to leave that relationship. This is a lot easier said than done because the abuser is usually manipulative (which is another sign of a toxic relationship). They can subtly attack you or disguise their abuse as love or affection. So, you may easily misconstrue their abuse and damage as love. But the truth is that you're being harmed by this relationship.

Moving on, a good way to stop toxic relationships is if nothing ever gets resolved. Every relationship will experience some rough patches, disagreements, and fights. However, in toxic relationships, these conflicts never get solved, as they simply end in arguments that don't productively address the issue. It could become a blame game, a screaming match, a guilt session, and so on. The communication in toxic relationships is such that you never get what you need out of a conversation. Aside from conflict resolution, you may also feel a lack when you're trying to confide in them. In a healthy relationship, both people share their struggles with each other and take turns supporting and being supported. But in toxic relationships, the focus will always be on the other person. It will never be your turn to be supported.

A partner in a toxic relationship will also not allow you any privacy. While it's good to be open and honest in a relationship, a bit of personal space and privacy is needed to maintain a healthy connection. But they may use guilt, shame, threats, and claims about trust to invade your privacy. This can be emotionally damaging for you. And in most cases, they maintain their right to privacy. They may be secretive about their life and not let you in. Finally, they may not even allow you the freedom to make your own decisions. In healthy relationships, big decisions are discussed together, and you each take the other's opinions, feelings, and preferences into account. This shows that you value each other. In toxic relationships, they may remove your autonomy from you and simply make all your decisions for you without asking you. This shows that they don't value you. So, if you're in a relationship that relates to any of these warning signs, you should reflect on how you can improve that relationship or (if all else fails) leave it.

Other than toxic relationships, there are also codependent relationships that can hinder your recovery process. During the development of your addiction, you may have formed some of these relationships. Codependency is related to imbalanced relationships, where one person enables the other person's self-destructive behavior (this can mean your addiction, poor mental health, irresponsibility, unhealthy habits, immaturity, and so on). Such relationships can be formed between you and a spouse, friend, partner, or even an employer. Codependency can be understood as relationship addiction. It's a behavioral and emotional condition that prevents you from forming a healthy and mutually satisfying relationship. Codependent relationships are often one-sided, emotionally destructive, or abusive. Codependent individuals can have good intentions, but their actions can be compulsive and unhealthy.

Signs of codependency are a desire to feel needed and actions made to rescue or support a loved one (you) that only lead them to become more dependent on them. Codependent individuals may act as martyrs and spend all their time caring for others.

This may lead them to lose sight of their own needs and wants, often causing harm to themselves and others. Examples of codependency in parent-child relationships can look like the parent doing everything for their adult child who should already be independent, the parent feeling a sense of meaning or purpose by forever financially supporting their adult child, the parent never allowing the child to do anything independently, and the child neglecting everything to respond to their parent's demands. In romantic relationships, codependency can look like investing a lot of time and energy into caring for the other person's addiction, making excuses for the other person's unhealthy habits or bad behavior, neglecting self-care to care for the other person, enabling the other person's destructive or unhealthy behavior (sometimes in an effort to keep them dependent on them), not allowing the other person to be independent, and not allowing the other person to take responsibility for their own actions and life.

If these signs apply to any of your relationships, then you must make an effort to stop being codependent. One way to do this is to look for signs of a healthy relationship. In order to forge a healthier relationship, you must understand what a healthy and loving relationship looks like. This will help you direct your relationship better. Signs of a healthy relationship include spending enough time together and apart (the exact amount of time for each will vary from person to person, so it's important to communicate and find a healthy balance), maintaining independence, being honest and open, having equality, and showing affection (again, each person gives and receives affection differently, so be sure to communicate how each of you shows affection). Another way to stop being codependent is to have healthy boundaries. While it's good to support each other, you must still respect each other's boundaries, as sometimes support is not needed or wanted. A boundary sets a clear limit for the other person to know what you're willing and unwilling to accept in a relationship. So, take some time and reflect on what's acceptable to you. Then, practice declining requests that step over your boundaries. It's not enough to have limits, you also need to enforce them. Finally, work on your self-esteem. Often, people in codependent relationships don't value or trust themselves. Therefore, invest some time in learning more about yourself and overcoming your negative self-talk.

On a related note, enabling relationships can also harm your recovery. Codependent relationships are often also enabling relationships, though not always. Enabling can take on many forms. They may make excuses, lie, or cover up for you when you exhibit unhealthy habits. These actions prevent you from facing the negative consequences of your actions, thus encouraging you to continue with your unhealthy habits since there were no negative outcomes. Such relationships are terrible for your recovery, as you will be encouraged to continue with your addiction.

Now that you know the relationships you can work on, leave, or avoid, let's turn our attention to how you can improve the healthy relationships that you do have. A lot of the time, your loved ones may want to support you during recovery, but they may not know how. Their efforts may often have the opposite effect. Their intentions may be pure, but they may not know how to approach, treat, or help you with your addiction. So, to help you help them (and to help them help you), let's explore how you can teach them to understand and approach your addiction.

The first thing to get out of the way is blame. Your loved ones may often think of your addiction and feel a component of self-blame. You may even feel like blaming others and your circumstances for your addiction. But this is simply not true. It's not their fault that you became addicted. Try to emphasize this to them and to yourself. If it helps, you can go back to the risk factors discussed in Chapter 2 to help you understand what contributed to your development of an addiction. The next thing to tell your loved ones is to not take things personally. When you're addicted to something, you may display several negative, unhealthy, and hurtful behaviors, such as lying, making false promises to never do things again, lashing out, and so on. It's easy for your loved ones to be affected by such actions and to take it personally. They may think that you wouldn't act in those ways if you really loved them. So, it's important to tell them that once addiction has a hold of you, your brain chemistry may change, and you may lose a bit of control over your actions and choices. It's not that you don't love them, it's just that your addiction sometimes colors your choices. They can try to not take things personally as much, and you can try to focus on recovery so that you partake in fewer of those hurtful behaviors.

Something else that can help your loved ones help you is for them to know when to take a step back. In their fervent desire to help you get better, they may end up feeling lonely and frustrated. They may overemphasize their role in your recovery and thus feel like there's always something more that they could be doing. But the reality is that they only play a supporting role in your recovery. It's an important role, but it's not the main one. The onus is on you to get better and keep moving forward. So, to prevent them from wrecking themselves trying to improve or progress your recovery, remind them that you're doing the work, and that their support is more than enough. On the subject of taking a step back, your loved ones must also understand that you may need outside help. Addictions can be chronic and fatal, so they may often require professional treatment. No matter your loved ones' expertise or knowledge, you will benefit more from professionals who have experience treating addiction. Even if it's not professionals, you may find support and comfort in others, such as other recovering addicts. This may make your family and loved ones feel useless or neglected. With that being said, it's good to explain to them how talking with others who have the same experiences and struggles as you can help you and facilitate your recovery.

A common mistake that your loved ones may make when approaching your addiction is to give you too much grace and acceptance. It's totally okay for them to not accept unacceptable behavior. And when you're dealing with addiction, you may display a wide range of such behavior. If they simply accept it, this may become an enabling relationship that reinforces your addiction due to the lack of consequences for your unhealthy habits and actions. Your loved ones may brush off certain undesirable behavior, thinking that you're simply going through the motions of your recovery or that the behavior is coming from your addiction rather than you. But making such excuses will only allow those undesirable behaviors to worsen. Rather than accepting any and all behavior (leading to enabling relationships), tell your loved ones to call you out on your unhealthy habits and to hold you accountable for your actions. Certain behaviors are simply unacceptable and your loved ones should have the freedom to voice out when your actions are hurting them. On a related note, it's healthy for them to have reasonable expectations of you. What may seem reasonable to them might be totally unreasonable when it comes to someone like you, who's dealing with an addiction. So, it's important to communicate in order to figure out where you're at in your recovery phase, so that your loved ones can understand what you're experiencing now and adjust their expectations accordingly. This is quite vital, as expectations that are too high may make you feel lousy about yourself and may make them feel frustrated or disappointed. Expectations that are too low may make them become complacent, accepting too little from you, and may make you lazy and unmotivated to do more. But when their expectations align with what you can push yourself to do, it can motivate you to keep moving forward, help you feel a sense of accomplishment, and help them feel happier in their relationship with you.

Next, remind your loved ones to focus on the present. They may get hung up on how your addiction developed in the first place or how it will affect your and their future. These concerns can distract them from focusing on your situation as it exists today. And your condition may be in constant flux, so this distraction can prevent them from really being present with you and supporting you. Finally, emphasize to your loved ones that, while their support and help is needed and appreciated, they should primarily be taking care of themselves. You shouldn't become the main focus in their lives. Everyone needs to take care of themselves before they can sustainably take care of others. So, just as you're focusing on healing yourself, they must focus on taking care of themselves. Just as you need a loving support system, they must also make sure that they're surrounding themselves with healthy relationships that support and comfort them. It can be stressful and emotionally distressing to have a loved one going through addiction. Make sure that their emotions and needs are being acknowledged and met.

Continuing the Battle

You've now reached the end of this book, and hopefully you feel more prepared to face and overcome your addiction. Along the way, if you ever need to refresh your memory on any given topic or treatment method, feel free to return to this book and flip to the area of interest. To help guide you, and as a little reminder on all that you've gained from this book, let's recap what each chapter touched on.

Chapter 1 explained what addiction is, and the symptoms you experience during addiction. Chapter 2 then expanded on what may happen before and after an addiction. That is, you studied the risk factors that make you more likely to develop an addiction and the negative effects that you face after falling into addiction. Chapter 3 started you on one of the commonly used methods of therapy for addiction: cognitive behavioral therapy (CBT). You learned what it is, how it works, and the benefits you can gain from it. CBT is based on the assumption that your psychological issues come from your thoughts and cognition, so it strives to correct them. In addition to gaining more understanding on CBT, you were also guided through SMART goal setting, case formulation, and other exercises that can help you develop the skills of CBT. In Chapter 4, you learned about another form of therapy that can be used to treat addiction: acceptance and commitment therapy (ACT). You discovered the various components of this therapy and how it can work to combat your addiction. ACT can be used to improve how you deal with negative situations. Rather than decreasing the frequency of your negative thoughts or urges, ACT can help you accept them and consciously choose to not indulge in them. The practices of ACT that you were led through are cognitive defusion, value clarification, and mindfulness.

Next, in Chapter 5, you studied yet another form of therapy, and that was exposure and response prevention (ERP) therapy. You explored the two components of this therapy and how they function to treat addiction. Then, you studied how to create a trigger ladder to help you confront and resist your triggers. In Chapter 6, you grew to understand relapses more, along with their potential causes, and how to prevent them. And lastly in Chapter 7, you realized how to spot negative, harmful relationships and how to build healthier ones during your recovery.

You've received a wealth of technical and practical knowledge that will help you as you recover from your addiction. Now that you have all this knowledge, remember to make full use of it. Apply the knowledge to your daily life in order to change your thoughts and behavior, as well as to increase your self-understanding and self-compassion. As a final parting word, it's relevant to emphasize the importance of being kind to yourself. When you're healing from addiction, it's easy to fall into self-destructive and self-critical behaviors. There's no end to the possible negative emotions that you will have to face. But as you're confronting all of that, it's important that you stay kind to yourself. Understand that what you're going through is difficult, and treat yourself the same way you would treat a friend. If you're able to be kind to yourself, you will be able to sustain your recovery and continue progressing.

References

Ackerman, C. (2017, March). *How does acceptance and commitment therapy (ACT) work?* PositivePsychology.com. https://positivepsychology.com/act-acceptance-and-commitment-therapy/

Ackerman, C. (2019, July 4). *25 CBT techniques and worksheets for cognitive behavioral therapy.* PositivePsychology.com. https://positivepsychology.com/cbt-cognitive-behavioral-therapy-techniques-worksheets/

Addiction Center. (2019). *Cognitive behavioral therapy - Addiction center.* AddictionCenter. https://www.addictioncenter.com/treatment/cognitive-behavioral-therapy/

Buddy, T. (2021, January 27). *How your recovery benefits from developing healthy relationships.* Verywell Mind. https://www.verywellmind.com/developing-healthy-relationships-to-maintain-abstinence-69450

Cherry, K. (2021). *Cognitive behavioral therapy.* Verywell Mind. https://www.verywellmind.com/what-is-cognitive-behavior-therapy-2795747

Dawn Rehab. (2018, June 29). *6 risk factors for addiction – How likely are you to become an addict?* The Dawn Wellness Centre and Rehab Thailand. https://thedawnrehab.com/blog/risk-factors-for-addiction/

Families for Addiction Recovery. (n.d.). *What are the risk factors?* Families for Addiction Recovery. https://www.farcanada.org/understanding-addiction/risk-factors/

Felman, A. (2018, October 26). *Addiction: Definition, symptoms, withdrawal, and treatment.* Www.medicalnewstoday.com. https://www.medicalnewstoday.com/articles/323465

Glasofer, D. (2015, October 29). *Acceptance and commitment therapy (ACT) for GAD.* Verywell Mind; Verywellmind. https://www.verywellmind.com/acceptance-commitment-therapy-gad-1393175

Guenzel, N., & McChargue, D. (2019, December 8). *Addiction relapse prevention.* Nih.gov; StatPearls Publishing. https://www.ncbi.nlm.nih.gov/books/NBK551500/

Huecker, M. R., Mohammadreza Azadfard, & Leaming, J. M. (2019, February 28). *Opioid addiction.* Nih.gov; StatPearls Publishing. https://www.ncbi.nlm.nih.gov/books/NBK448203/

International OCD Foundation. (2010). *International OCD Foundation | Exposure and Response Prevention (ERP).* International OCD Foundation. https://iocdf.org/about-ocd/ocd-treatment/erp/

McLean Hospital. (n.d.). *A guide to exposure and response prevention therapy | McLean Hospital.* Www.mcleanhospital.org. https://www.mcleanhospital.org/essential/erp

NHS. (2022, January 18). *Addiction: what is it?* Nhs.uk. https://www.nhs.uk/live-well/addiction-support/addiction-what-is-it/

OCD UK. (2018). *What is exposure response prevention (ERP)? | OCD-UK.* Ocduk.org. https://www.ocduk.org/overcoming-ocd/accessing-ocd-treatment/exposure-response-prevention/

Partnership to End Addiction. (n.d.). *Preventing teen drug use: Risk factors and why teens use.* Partnership to End Addiction | Where Families Find Answers. https://drugfree.org/article/risk-factors-problem-use-addiction/

Scott, E. (2018). *Can mindfulness relieve more than stress?* Verywell Mind. https://www.verywellmind.com/mindfulness-the-health-and-stress-relief-benefits-3145189

Scott, E. (2021, September 13). *Release tension with this targeted meditation technique.* Verywell Mind. https://www.verywellmind.com/body-scan-meditation-why-and-how-3144782

Sternlicht, L., & Sternlicht, A. (n.d.). *10 most common reasons for addiction relapse: Family addiction specialist: Addiction counselor.* Www.familyaddictionspecialist.com. https://www.familyaddictionspecialist.com/blog/10-most-common-reasons-for-addiction-relapse

Stibich, M. (2019). *How to make your health goals S.M.A.R.T.* Verywell Mind. https://www.verywellmind.com/smart-goals-for-lifestyle-change-2224097

Tyler, M. (2014). *Risk factors for addiction.* Healthline. https://www.healthline.com/health/addiction/risk-factors

Tyler, M. (2018, May 24). *What is addiction?* Healthline; Healthline Media. https://www.healthline.com/health/addiction

VitaNova. (2019, March 3). *11 surprising facts about addiction.* Vita Nova Rehab. https://vitanovarehab.com/blog/11-surprising-facts-addiction/